Gloria –
Thank you.
for touching the
lives of so many –
G♡ ... bless
PB

10 Feet
FROM THE EDGE
Stuck *in the* Comfort Zone

A story of survival and lessons on how shifting
our attitudes, making better choices, overcoming
fears and eliminating negative beliefs can move
us from stuck in our comfort zone to living life
with purpose, passion and possibility.

Peggy Brockman

Peggy Brockman

PB

Cover and Author Photography by **Callie Gardiner, Callie Gardiner Photography**
Cover and book design by **Kendra Cagle, 5 Lakes Design**
Cover Copy & Content Editing by **Julie Escobar, Speakers Choice Consulting**
Final Editing by **Kelly Humphrey**

Gloria —
Thank you, the
for living of this so warm,
God Bless!
Love, [signature]

ISBN-13:
978-1499100662

ISBN-10:
1499100663

FIRST EDITION
10 Feet from the Edge: Stuck in the Comfort Zone
Peggy Plummer Brockman

In Memory of:

Dr. Henry Laws and Chaplain Kenneth L. Bohannon who were with me at University Hospital in Birmingham, Alabama (UAB); my surgeon Dr. James Pollack; and dear friend and nurse from Palms of Pasadena Hospital in St. Petersburg, Florida, Peggy Pratt. You each touched so many lives while you were here in your earthly bodies. I know you continue to bless us as angels in heaven.

In Dedication and Appreciation of:

To Bill, my husband, to my girls Brooklyn, Callie, Tina, Jeanette and Stacy, and to my grandchildren Sydian, Elijah, Evan, Brock, Janine, Craig and Grace – You are my reason, my motivation and the loves of my life. I have learned so much from each of you.

My family and friends, you have been through the worst with me and encouraged me in times of need. What I have learned is that life is what we make of it – WE get to choose!

To my John Maxwell Team family – you helped me find my passion again and encouraged me to use the tools I've learned to add value to lives around the world.

Debbie Bean Ragan, Janie Matthews, Dr. Pete Weinheimer and all the nurses and doctors who were with me at UAB hospital in 1975-76 – you helped me through the most difficult time in my life. You will forever be in my heart.

To all nurses and doctors who add value to so many lives across the world – you are true heroes.

Table of Contents

"Some let a moment define them and hold them back. Some take control and define the moment using it to propel them forward."

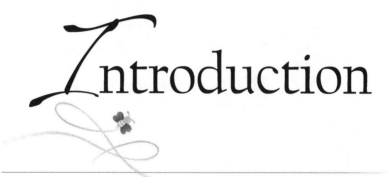ntroduction

Life is full of challenges. Things can be moving along smoothly then one day – in an instant – life changes forever. It happens to people everywhere. It can be an unexpected divorce, a sudden death, an accident, or in my case, an illness that changed my life forever.

When these things happen to us or someone we're close to, WE get to choose how we handle it. WE get to choose our attitude. Ever wonder why some choose to wallow in the self-pity for years and some are able to "put their big girl panties on" and move forward? It is because some let a moment define them and hold them back. Some take control and define the moment, using it to propel them forward.

Through the ups and downs in my life, I became a survivor. I learned to push through my fears, shift my attitude and let go of beliefs I formed about myself along the way.

You can do it too. In my book, *10 Feet from The Edge: Stuck in the Comfort Zone,* I will teach you how. As an author, speaker, trainer and coach, it is what I do. It is who I am: A survivor who lives life with passion, purpose and possibility and a mission to add value to all those I have the opportunity to reach.

Let me share a little insight on my family and where I came from so you will understand a little more of my life before you read my story and the lessons I have to share.

I was born in 1956 in Anniston, Alabama to Robert L. (Bob) and Jeanne Plummer. At almost the exact time I was born, an ammunition igloo exploded at Anniston Ordinance Depot, where my mother worked. I still have the telegram that was sent to my parents in the scrapbook of my life. Maybe THAT was a sign of things to come.

I was a precocious child – always into something. At the age of four, I quietly hid from the nanny until she panicked and called my parents. Then there was the time I decided to strip down at the neighborhood playground to wash my clothes in the mud puddle! Yes, I was always into something!

In high school, my classmates voted me Most Popular. Perhaps it was because of my all-inclusive nature – I always tried to be nice to everyone. I didn't like cliques that excluded other people. I found them unfair and dividing. We were all equal, right? We just came from different backgrounds and different life situations, but it didn't make us "better" than one another; it only created diversity and varied perspectives.

I grew up in Anniston, a small town in northeast Alabama. My family was what you would call upper middle class. Both my parents had good jobs and we had everything we needed and most of the time we had the extras we wanted. I am the baby of four. I have two sisters and a brother.

Donna is two years older than I, and I have always treasured our relationship. Even though she really hated me "borrowing" her clothes in high school, and has probably never forgiven me for spending her mercury head dime collection on candy at the YMCA, we have always maintained a special closeness for all we have shared over the years. I know without a doubt, Donna would be there for me at any time. I hope she knows the same about me.

Sharon, six years older than I, was definitely not my favorite sibling growing up. It may have been because she hated babysitting us (which she had to do so many times), and the truth is, I probably was not the most cooperative kid. We fought like cats and dogs! But now, as an adult, I can see that there are so many ways we are alike. They say you should look within if there is something you dislike so much about someone else – it just might be one of your own traits! Sharon and I share a lot of common interests and beliefs now and have a bond we found as adults that I am grateful for.

My brother, Tommy, is nine years older than I. He was the one who always liked to unsnap every one of our Velcro hair rollers at least once a week. He would spray Right Guard deodorant under our bedcovers then pull them over our head and hold them just to mess with us. We would scream at him then we would all laugh so hard. There was such a difference in our ages; we never had the opportunity to be close growing up. He's the one who made me an Auburn fan since, at the formative ages of thirteen to fifteen; I would occasionally go to his home in Auburn to spend weekends babysitting my niece.

Unfortunately, my brother recently experienced something similar to my story. For a couple of months, my family and I relived that horrific nightmare we had lived some 38 years before. Through this, I have come to know him better and begin to create a stronger bond and closeness between us. I thank God for giving us this time together as adults. We both narrowly escaped our own departure from this earth.

We were all basically good kids and we grew to be successful adults with families of our own. Our parents instilled good values in us that would follow us throughout our lives. Values we would pass to our children and grandchildren. Values I would draw on throughout my life in difficult times and in good times.

As you read my story of survival and the other stories I use to create the lessons in this book, I hope you will think about your own life and how you can use your story to make a difference in the lives of others. If you are struggling, caught up in your beliefs – your story – blaming others for your challenges, STOP. JUST STOP. Choose differently. Get out of your comfort zone – especially if it is one of 'poor, pitiful me'. Choose to take back your power and move forward in life with a positive attitude. My hope for you is that you learn to live your life with passion, purpose and possibility.

“*In life, our attitudes, choices, fears, and beliefs will always* determine our successes, *failures and degree of what I call 'stuckedness'.***”**

Chapter 1

The *Choices*
We Make
Define Our Lives

In life, our attitudes, choices, fears and beliefs will always determine our successes, failures and degree of what I call "stuckedness". At a very young age I learned to deal with fears – and about how the choices WE make play a major role in all facets of our lives. Later in life, I gained a deep understanding of how my beliefs would affect the big picture of who I am as a human being.

My early childhood was pretty normal, but at the age of 17, my life was forever changed. I remember the day very clearly. I went to the bathroom and the toilet was filled with blood. Looking back, I realized I had suffered with stomachaches on and off for several years, but this was noticeably different. My parents immediately took me in to see our family internal medicine doctor, who began trying to determine what was going on.

So the testing began. Unfortunately, this was before the practice of doing routine colonoscopies. Those of you from my generation might remember the procedure that proceeded colonoscopies – the dreaded metal proctoscope! Well, let me just tell you – there was no anesthesia. You were wide awake and it was NOT a pleasant experience. In fact, I would put it in the horrific category for a young girl the age of 17.

For those of you who might not have had the experience, I will spare you the graphic details, but just imagine the painful experience of being belly down and knees folded with your shoulders pressed firmly against the surface of the table as air is pumped through your intestinal tract. Well you know, what goes in must come out – and that is NOT something a good southern girl ever thinks will be OK! There is only ONE attitude you can have about that and it is NOT a good one!

Well, after thorough review it was determined I had what could be a very debilitating disease – ulcerative colitis, a disease of the large intestine also known as the colon. I was given all types of harsh drugs and forced into what I called "the mushy food diet" – not at all what I wanted to be eating at 17 years old! I definitely needed an attitude adjustment after that visit. This was hard.

I got really stuck in that place of anger and feeling sorry for myself. I liked the comfort of my life as it was before. I didn't want to accept that I was sick with a disease that might never go away. I was feeling the pain of uncertainty. I knew this was something I had to live with – but as a lively teenager I didn't want to settle. I had the opportunity to really look at myself and my life and make a choice about how I was going to deal with this. I suddenly found myself thrust into growing up really fast and having to make some tough choices. These choices would dictate the future of my wellbeing.

Because of the constant loss of blood, the medications and just the disease itself, my low energy level no longer allowed me to continue some of the activities I once loved. I had been a cheerleader since elementary school and now, going into my senior (and most important) high school year, I had to face the reality that my body was not healthy enough to endure the strenuous physical strain this put on me. I had to make the choice to give up cheerleading. It was painful. It had been a huge part of my life but (even though it felt like it for a moment) it was not the end of the world. It was a choice I had to make for my health.

Since it was much less strenuous, I continued my modeling career, putting more focus on that and telling myself it would be better anyway since I had lost so much weight. My illness was debilitating, and I lived with the burden of that at a very young age. There were days I felt great! Then, of course, I'd do what teens do, and make a foolish choice like eating pizza and drinking soda. Of course that was soon followed with me being doubled over in pain and being violently ill for a few days.

But you know, sometimes I made that choice. It was less about being willful and more about being NORMAL. To fit in at a party with friends. To just be a kid. I remember once going to Fort Walton Beach, Florida, where I live now, the summer after my high school graduation with my best friend, Annette. All I wanted was to experience what I believed all new graduates deserved!

In Florida, we were old enough to buy beer and Boone's Farm Strawberry Wine, so we did. We also bought pizza and every other kind of junk food you can imagine. And, believe me, I paid for it – and not just in dollars. I still remember lying on the bed doubled over in excruciating pain, just praying that I wouldn't die, yet at the same time thinking how much better it would feel if I did. I was suffering from my own CHOICES because I was stuck in the zone of wanting to be a "normal" teenager.

Over the next year or so I learned to manage my disease. I just kept pushing through. I was in college, working at "The Withit" junior clothing store and planning my wedding. I guess I didn't really slow down until that day when my body started screaming at me, "Nope! That's it! You're in BIG trouble now!" Four weeks after the big wedding and honeymoon in the summer of '75, I was on what felt like my death bed. I just didn't realize how close to the truth that feeling was. I would lie in bed with a trashcan by my head and would crawl to the bathroom when I could manage it. I couldn't keep anything down except French vanilla pudding with bananas and vanilla wafers. I remember lying in the bed eating it by the bowlful. It became my "comfort food." At least it tasted the same going down as it did coming up!

When I finally went to the local hospital it was almost too late. They tried to pull me through it, but the disease was too advanced. I was taken to University Hospital in Birmingham, Alabama, to a specialist in colorectal surgery. For the next couple of days they fed me anything I would eat to try to build up my system enough to endure the surgery I was about to undergo.

I began to learn what it meant to be a patient in a teaching hospital. Talk about some of the most embarrassing moments in life! I got to REALLY check my attitude my first couple of days at UAB. Remember the proctoscope story? Yep, the doc and five male medical school students (ALL not much older than I) in the room for that one. I CHOOSE to laugh about it now, but it remains one of those difficult choices since it was truly humiliating at the time.

The doctors feared if they waited any longer my colon might rupture, so the decision was made to do surgery to remove my colon – all of my large intestines. I soon found out that meant I would have something called a stoma. A stoma is where they bring the small intestine up to the stomach wall to create an opening to eliminate the waste. I would wear a bag on my stomach for the rest of my life to cover that hole and collect the feces. You really get to choose your attitude when you hear something like that.

So many thoughts and questions were running through my head. I am only 19 years old. I had only been married for six weeks. I can only imagine the fear and struggle my young husband was suffering through. At the ripe old age of 21, all of a sudden, his world – our world – was completely upside down. Why me? Why this? Will I ever be able to go swimming again? What about my modeling? Will my husband still want me? So many thoughts and questions began pouring through my head.

The next day a really cheerful woman walked into my room. She was very attractive and well dressed. She introduced herself and began to explain to me that she was from the local Ostomy Association, and she wanted to come by to see if I had any questions about the surgery I was about to have. She explained that she, too, had the same surgery several years earlier. Her message was simple. "You and your body will go through a big change. Although it is a permanent change, it will be OK." In fact, she went on to explain, "You can live a pretty normal life." Then she added the most important thing: "IF YOU CHOOSE TO."

She let me know that I could choose to wallow in self-pity and be miserable or I could choose to live my life fully and be a testament to others who suffer through challenges like mine. She had lived a normal, full life, so why couldn't I? I truly appreciated the calm she brought to me and to my family in the short time she spent visiting my bedside.

My young mind was racing through the minutes and hours of those days just before surgery, and this was the time in my life where that positive attitude I had always been known for needed to find its way home. The questions just kept flying through my mind. Would I be able to have sex again? Will I be able to have children? What about the gymnastics I loved doing? Would I smell bad with this bag collecting my poop? What if it burst open or leaked?

OH MY GOD, WHAT IS HAPPENING TO ME?

But I kept hearing her calm words…

you will be ok…
you will live a normal life.

IF YOU CHOOSE TO.

The morning of surgery Dr. Henry Laws, my beloved surgeon, showed up with his boyish energy and said "Ms. P (as he lovingly called me), I have an idea! There is a new procedure called the Kock Pouch. I haven't done one yet but I have studied it and I am confident I can. What we will do is build an internal pouch or collection reservoir out of the healthy intestines. You will still have a stoma like a regular ileostomy, but it will be tiny and it will be low enough on your belly you can still wear a bikini! Best thing is – you won't have to wear an external bag. You will just insert a catheter in to the stoma and drain the pouch. What do you think?"

I can still see him sitting in that chair by my bed brimming with confidence. "NOW THAT'S MORE LIKE IT!" I thought to myself. "I can live with that!" So my family and I discussed it and made the decision to move forward with the Kock Pouch procedure.

The day of surgery was a long one for my family. Surgery was over nine hours long, and the days that followed would be even longer and harder. I was a woman of faith and it was my faith, my family and my friends that pulled me through the days that followed what turned out to be the first surgery.

The complications were many and the struggles seemed endless. I developed an intestinal blockage so they put a tube with a mercury ball on the end down my nose that could work its way in to my intestinal tract. Hopefully this would break up that blockage. They decided to insert a central line in the subclavian vein so they could feed the hyperalimentation formula (or super nutrient formula) through my veins to sustain my nutritional system and build me up. It was mandatory: no solid food.

My family and I really liked Dr. B, the senior resident, at that time. He was a good doctor and he would be the one to insert the "hyper-a" line. I had to sign a waiver due to the fact that it was possible during this procedure to puncture the lung, but he had never had that happen so I should not be concerned. It seems that was the beginning of things to come. After the catheter was inserted, I made the trip to the X-ray room to make sure everything was positioned properly.

Bad news again. My lung had been punctured in the process, and as a result it deflated. I spent many more hours in the X-ray area over the next several days, weeks and what became months. To this day, I still get a sick feeling every time I get close enough to an X-ray area that I can smell the chemicals.

With a deflated lung I was dependent on oxygen to breathe. The next thing that happened was a fluid build-up in the lung. They had to insert a drain tube in my side between two ribs to relieve that issue. This happened a couple more times over the next few very long weeks. Eventually, the blockage in my intestines broke through and I was able to eat very soft foods. But I must admit – to this day the very thought of eating cherry gelatin ever again makes me nauseated.

The day finally came to learn how to insert the catheter into the stoma on my abdomen to drain the pouch. I will never forget it! I was certainly apprehensive, and so was my favorite nurse, Debbie. In fact, as I later found out, she was scared to death! She didn't show it that day – it was her job and she did it with confidence. We connected recently after 38 years and it was one of the things we reminisced about. Dr. Laws handed her the catheter and said go put this in and drain the pouch! They had inserted a mushroom catheter in the pouch to keep the valve open so there would not be any back pressure on it while I had the blockage. That had to be removed first. She was so afraid she was going to puncture something but she was a true pro. She took a deep breath, walked in with confidence, and said "Let's do this!" It's definitely something we can laugh about today!

Six weeks after my original surgery I was finally going home! They had taught me how to insert the catheter myself. I could have independence with this new way of eliminating my body's waste, and I could care for my own personal hygiene. I am here to tell you, it is a weird experience when you first insert a 12-inch catheter into a hole in your stomach that shouldn't be there! That couple of days before I left the hospital, I wasn't feeling stellar. I made one of the most foolish choices of my life – way worse than the pizza and beer. I don't know that I have shared this with anyone to this day, but I'm about to share it with you dear reader …. my dirty, dark secret.

66 The choices we make in life can define the rest of our lives. I made a stupid young mistake.

A really bad choice

And it could've cost me my life. 99

Chapter 2

My *Dirty* Dark Secret

This is one of those choices in life that defined my future and almost took my life. It is really hard to admit that I was so foolish. I can make the excuse that I was young, that I was desperate. All "those" things we tell ourselves when we know we are making a detrimental choice. There is no turning back now, so I will just lay it out there. It actually feels good to just cleanse it from my soul.

I began to run a low-grade temperature, and I was so desperate to go home, I would actually take the thermometer out of my mouth if they walked out of the room or turned around. This way it wouldn't register that I had a fever. After all, it was just low grade – barely even considered a fever. Probably from the excitement of going home, I convinced myself.

The choices we make in life can define the rest of our lives. I can't turn the clock back, and maybe it would not have made a difference anyway, but it was foolish and it was dangerous.

My temp SHOWED normal that day, so we packed up my bags and off we went back to Anniston. They had told my family that I might experience some depression dealing with the ostomy surgery and the change in my body, and that they shouldn't buy into it. Good advice IF that is actually what I had been experiencing.

As the week after returning home progressed, I became weaker and weaker. My new husband and I were staying at my parent's home so they could help take care of me. I remember my mother calling me to dinner one night. I was back in the bedroom lying down since I wasn't feeling so well. I got up to attempt to go to the kitchen, but my legs were so weak I knew I was not going to make it. I called for help, but they were not going to give in to my helplessness as they had been warned this might happen.

I remember gripping the wall and slinking down into the hallway. Unable to get up, I watched down the long hall through the den into the kitchen as they all gathered around the table to eat. If I wanted to eat, I would get up and come in there. You see, they didn't know my dirty little secret about the fever.

I had been home about a week and my parents were finally able to go somewhere – it had been a long couple of months of hospital sitting and driving back and forth the 50-plus miles to get there. They went to an Alabama football game where my sister Donna was attending college. I remember the day just like it was yesterday. It's so clear and vivid in my mind.

I was lying on the gold couch in the den watching television. I had grown weaker and weaker as each day passed, but I was determined to push through and not let this lick me. I mustered up the strength to stand up and walk around the circular coffee table. As I stood up a white liquid began to pour out of me, running down my legs. I called my doctor and I remembered telling him I thought I was trying to start my period or something. What I don't remember telling him was that my fever was now up to 102 degrees.

Later that evening my parents came home. I am sure it had

been such a relief to just get out and have some fun away from the caretaking. I was so happy for them. As the evening rolled on, it became apparent that my fever was rising. At 2:00 a.m., an ambulance came to pick me up at my parent's home to take me back to University Hospital in Birmingham. My fever was 106 degrees by now and my body was going into shock.

To this day, every time I see an ambulance I have a flashback of that night. In the dark of the night, in the wee hours of the morning, all I could remember was seeing the red lights of the ambulance flash on the road signs as we roared down the highway. I was so sick I thought I was going to die. I just didn't know how close I was. Each time I threw up, I prayed, and prayed hard. I begged God to give me another day. Even though a small part of me thought dying would be easier, I just wanted to live.

I made a stupid young mistake. A really bad choice. And it could've cost me my life. I had so much to live for. "Please don't let me die," I cried. It is hard to write these words. All the pain and fear that I felt that night has been stuffed deep inside and remembering it brings it all back. The pain I caused my family and my friends. I just wanted the nightmare I was living to be over. I just wanted to go home and be a young, happy newlywed. Didn't I deserve that?

Dr. Laws was away at a medical conference, but Dr. Pete Weinheimer (Dr. Pete, as I so fondly called him), my favorite senior resident, was waiting on me in the emergency room. He struggled to get a tube down my nose and into my stomach to help relieve the nausea. I can still remember the frustration I could see on his face, and I sensed a sort of desperation as he knew how critical I was. He had spent a lot of time in my room caring for me and he wasn't going to lose me now. I believe he saved my life that night.

They brought in an ice mattress to try to lower my temperature, and they pumped me full of cortisone to help bring my body out of the shock it was in. Blood work and X-rays showed I had a serious infection. I had a fistula, a hole in the intestinal surgery site, so the feces had been draining into my abdomen for who knows how long. By now I had developed peritonitis and the poison ran throughout my blood stream. I had abscessed through my abdominal wall and through my female organs so badly, the infection drained vaginally that day when I stood up. My grandmother had died from peritonitis just six years before. I knew this and so did the rest of my family. Would I die, too?

They spent the next 24 hours just trying to stabilize me in hopes I could hold out until Dr. Laws could get there. He was in constant contact by phone but the surgery had to happen now. It couldn't wait. I couldn't wait. My life depended on it.

Dr. Pete and Dr. Laws called in another specialist and off to surgery I went. They opened me back up and washed and cleaned out all the infection they could. They found the fistula and repaired it. My family waited in sheer agony, not knowing if I could survive this or not. I went from surgery to the Intensive Care Unit as they still had me on a breathing tube and they needed to make sure I was being watched very closely.

I remember waking up in there with this big breathing tube down my throat and feeling like I was choking on it. I remember the man who was right across from me screaming out in agony after he was brought in from a car accident. And I remember his family crying out in pain when he didn't survive it.

I wanted out of there and I wrote that on a note. I needed my family with me. They were my strength and I needed them now to hold my hand and to assure me it would be OK and that I would survive this nightmare. The doctors understood, so they moved me to a regular room with a 24-hour nurse, and my family sat there with me 24/7. My mother would stay with me during the day. She would keep everyone hopping and making sure I had everything I needed.

My young husband rotated between days and nights, but my daddy would stay most nights. He seemed to be the one who could calm me the most. I owe him a thousand plus foot rubs still to this day for all the nights he sat and rubbed my feet. It was the only thing that would calm me. I remember him taking his tie and tying one end to his foot and one end to my hand so if I needed him I could just pull the tie while he attempted to sleep. If he hadn't been with me that one night, I probably wouldn't be here today.

The girl from the blood lab had come in earlier that day to draw blood. It was always a game to see who could succeed in getting blood as my veins were virtually non-existent for blood drawing and they were constantly doing it. Back then they didn't do all the stuff they do now to make that easier!

She couldn't find a vein in my arm so she made an almost fatal decision to draw blood from my foot. Bad choice. I had been so immobile that I threw a blood clot to my leg that traveled rapidly to my lung. Daddy knew something was wrong and he insisted the nurses run tests. They were able to stop it before it went to my heart, which would have been an immediate death sentence.

Three days later, my temperature was up again and something wasn't right. Dr. Laws and Dr. Pete came into my room together after the X-rays were taken, and I knew by the look on their faces it was not good news. Dr. Laws kind of shook his head and he said "Ms. P, we've got to go back in. There is another abscess." I could see the pain on his face. We had become quite close.

During surgery, they opened me up from just under my breast down as far as they could go so they could once again flush out the abdominal cavity in hopes of preventing any more infection. They had to break my rib cage to get to the abscess. They packed the incision with gauze and left it open to heal from the inside out. There were these three-inch rubber tubes that were stitched to each side crossing the incision to hold it in place. The pain of trying to move took my breath away as my rib cage healed. I dreaded the moments the nurses would come in my room and tell me they were going to sit me up on the side of the bed. I had to have an oxygen mask to breathe. I was living my hell. But at least I was living.

❝You can choose to give up, to die and take all the hopes, dreams and talents God has given you with you. Or you can choose to live and use all those talents and lessons learned through this experience to add value — to

make a difference

in the lives of others.❞

- CHAPLAIN KENNETH L. BOHANNON
University Hospital, Birmingham, AL
1975

Chapter 3

10 *Feet* from the *Edge*

There was that one day where I just couldn't fight the fight any longer. I was done. I wanted to give up because I couldn't understand why all this kept happening to me. What had I done so wrong that God would put me and my family through this? I felt so guilty for everything my family was going through.

My sister Donna had been there for me through some of the hardest times, and she gave me such strength. She would come up from college as often as she could. She was there when they put the lung tube in, and she didn't flinch as I squeezed her hands so tightly. She held me as I sobbed on her shoulder and talked about how tired I was of it all. I just wanted all the pain to stop. I could be honest with her. She was not only my sister; she was my friend. She wasn't much older than I was and it was a heavy burden for her to bear as well. I am forever grateful to her for being there for me.

My new husband and his family, my family, they had all been there around the clock trying to balance traveling between Anniston and Birmingham with work and life. It was physically and emotionally draining on all of them watching me go through this and living the nightmare with me. We were two and a half months into this hell and had no idea when it would end.

They did everything they could to keep my spirits up. Forrest, my husband's uncle, was always the jokester and always doing all he could to make me laugh in spite of the circumstances surrounding us. I remember how, before I went home, he talked about that one day he was really worried. The one day I told him I didn't know if I was going to make it.

I was in excruciating pain, I was scared and I was questioning everything about my life. Would this be all there was for me for the rest of my living days? Would my life ever have real meaning or would I just be a burden on all those who loved and cared for me? Not only was the physical pain almost more than I could bear, the emotional pain was just as bad. My life was hanging on by a thread. I was 10 feet from the edge of giving up.

Chaplain Bohannon, the hospital chaplain, was a regular visitor to my room. He spent many days visiting my bedside and he always had insightful words of wisdom for me. He was there that one day I was ready to give up. He sat by my bed and held my hand as he spoke of the only power I had left:

The *power* of CHOICE.

He lovingly looked at me and said, "Peggy, I understand that you are tired and that you want to give up. Today you have a choice and it will be the biggest choice of your life. You can choose to give up, to die and take all the hopes, dreams and talents God has given you with you. Or you can choose to live and use all those talents and lessons learned through this experience to add value and to make a difference in the lives of others. But if you choose to live, you will choose to live with the emotional and physical scars this battle has left upon you. Each and every day of your life you will get to choose your attitude with which you will deal with this. It is your choice. I hope you choose to live.

Your family and your friends hope you choose to live, however, your choice is the only one that matters."

That was almost 40 years ago. I will be forever grateful to the good chaplain. He will never know the impact he had on my life and continues to have on the lives of so many others as a result of that conversation.

For the next few months I fought for my life every day. I was determined to get out of that bed and walk out of that hospital. I went four months without a solid bite of food. I had to learn to walk again due to muscle atrophy. At 5'8" tall, I weighed 85 pounds at one time. My daddy could touch his finger and thumb together around my leg above my knee. But I survived, and five and a half months after that first surgery, I walked out of University Hospital alive and determined to thrive again, and to add value to the lives of others.

I was so blessed that God had answered my prayers and the prayers of so many others. He let me live a full life and even give birth to two beautiful children. After the abscess had penetrated my female organs, they said I would never have children because of all the scar tissue. They were wrong. God had his own plan in my life.

I have so many people to be thankful for during that whole ordeal. Not only was my family there, but my husband and his family were there and all my close friends from high school were there. I spent six of the first seven months of my marriage in the hospital. The first Halloween, Thanksgiving, Christmas,

New Year's and Valentine's Day were spent in the hospital.

I will always remember the week before Christmas.

My mother, who was quite persuasive, convinced the hospital staff to let her set up a big Christmas tree, lights and all, in my room. She knew Christmas was one of my favorite holidays and she wanted to add just a little joy to my life. She wanted me to smile again.

Shortly after that, my sister Donna came to see me. She was trying her best to talk me into putting on some make-up and exchanging that ugly blue hospital gown for my own night gown "so I would feel better." She had brought a couple dozen cookies, too, which I couldn't have. I should have suspected something but I didn't feel well enough that day to even care or notice.

Suddenly William, one of my best friends from elementary school, popped his head in the door and said, "Hi Peggy, I just wanted to pop in and say hello!" Then he disappeared. Next came Vaughn, then Pat and Paula, and Jacob, and many others repeating the process. One by one they filed passed my room popping their heads in, waving, saying hello and then leaving. At the end of that line, my junior high school boyfriend, Gary, came in my room with a big, "HO, HO, HO!" He was dressed as Santa Claus carrying a big pack of gifts over his back. More than 15 of my friends filed in to my hospital room after Santa, and it was a joyous day.

It is one of my favorite memories of that time, and each of these friends is so special to me for being there. They had all piled in a big van and driven over to see me. It was the oddest assortment of people from my high school. People who normally would not have hung out together necessarily, but they were all there together and it made me happy. Now I knew why my sister wanted me to put on the make-up and gown, which, of course, I had NOT done! That one act of kindness gave me the energy and the drive to push through, and I was no longer depressed about being in the hospital for Christmas.

The day I was told I would get to go home in the next week or two was a big day of celebration. It happened to be my six month wedding anniversary, and it was the first time I ate a "real" meal. The hospital staff fixed us steak and baked potatoes and rolled it in on a silver cart. Well, a stainless cart, along with a small celebration cake. The Birmingham News, the local paper, was there to take pictures and write a story and I was in my fanciest night gown.

I was skinny as a rail, had lost most of my hair and my face was round and "moon faced" from all the steroids, but I was beautiful. Life was beautiful. I was beautiful because I was alive and because I had become a different person while going through this life-altering experience. I had begun to fully understand the meaning of living a values-based life. I understood at such a deep level the true meaning of friendship and family. I knew the power of choice and the importance of having a good attitude and believing in something, someone, bigger than me. I had a level of maturity that only an experience like this could create.

Over the next several days after the celebration, the nurses would come by to celebrate the fact I would be going home, and one by one they shared their stories of the days they left for their days off and never expected me to be there when they returned. It was a success story of survival for them, too. They were responsible for my recovery and had cared for me all those days and nights. They had cried with me and celebrated with me and now I would finally go home for good to start my life over again. It would be a new life, a new normal. I was so blessed to have that new opportunity for that new normal, knowing what I had faced and how close I had come to never having a chance at any normal.

Because I still had a fistula, I would continue to need to keep the mushroom catheter in to keep the pouch flowing freely. That meant I would need to continue wearing the external bag I had been wearing to collect the feces. I could handle it – but I was scared.

The hospital had become my new comfort zone. There I had all the trained nurses and doctors to take care of me. At home, I would have to do it all on my own, and that was frightening. I knew I could do it. I was a smart young adult, right? But what if the bag leaked? What if it filled with air and exploded? "What if's" filled my thoughts.

I chose to focus on the fact I was so grateful to be alive, I didn't care. It wasn't what I chose for myself, but it was what life had dealt me and I had to believe it was for a reason. This was for the rest of my life. This was my new normal and I realized I was the only one who could choose my attitude, so I chose to make it a positive one! This was my first real step in healing and moving forward.

66 *Sometimes our comfort zone might not be a*

'comfortable' place,

*yet it is all we know and so we, in some
sort of way, thrive in it. We talk about it all the
time and we perpetuate it being what it is.* 99

Chapter 4

Living
the Lessons

One thing that would help me move forward was getting creative with covering the bag that hung on my body. My daddy ran a sewing factory, so I had him make me some covers out of fancy material. I had red satin with a black satin heart on it, I had animal print ones, and when I became pregnant, I had a pink one that said "It's a girl" because I wanted a girl. I began visiting other people at my local hospital who were going through the same thing, just as the woman had done for me. I shared stories of hope and survival and living. I reminded them they would no longer be doubled over in pain every day and they wouldn't have to be afraid to go somewhere due to the constant diarrhea. I helped them believe they could deal with the other stuff. After all, I had.

I remember one call in particular I received from the hospital. A woman was very ill and was at that point that removing her colon had become an emergency, yet she refused to have the surgery. She had created all these scenarios in her mind about how horrible life would be for her if she had ostomy surgery. She was giving into her fears of the beliefs she had created in her mind. She actually thought that just going ahead and dying would be better.

I walked into her room with a smile on my face and introduced myself. I told her I had received a call from her doctor asking me to just come by and visit with her to discuss any questions she might have about having ostomy surgery. She looked straight at me and said "Well you might as well leave then because I am not having that surgery. I would rather die."

Knowing how hard I had fought to live, I almost lost my cool, but I didn't. I looked straight at her and asked her what she was afraid of. She began to list all her fears. She talked about how she would never be able to go out of her house again, how she would never be able to eat the foods she had always loved, she wouldn't be able to wear nice clothes again, etc. I had to chuckle. Here I was standing there in her room in my nice clothes and I had an ostomy.

I asked her how long it had been since she had been out of her home. She told me it had been over a year because she never knew when she would have diarrhea. I asked her how long it had been since she had been able to eat the foods she had loved. She said it had been at least three years. I just looked in her eyes and calmly said, "I am here, standing in your room, wearing my nice clothes and I just had a big lunch of barbeque chicken, potato salad and baked beans. I take gymnastics and I teach swimming. I live the life I am so blessed to have been gifted. AND, I have an ostomy bag. So, I am going to share something with you that someone said to me at this point in my life. Today you get to make a choice. You can live if you choose to or you can give up and die. It is your choice. I hope you choose to live and live life to the fullest. I will hold your hand through it if that is what you need."

She looked at me for a long moment, rolled over and picked up the phone and called her doctor and said, "Schedule me for surgery in the morning."

You see, she was living in the comfort zone of sickness and self-pity, and change was frightening. Sometimes our comfort zone might not be a "comfortable" place, yet it is all we know and so we, in some sort of way, thrive in it. We talk about it all the time and we perpetuate it being what it is. Sometimes we even use it as an excuse to not do more or to not do things we simply don't want to do or are afraid to do.

We know what it is like right here in this place, no matter how broken or dysfunctional it is, yet we don't know what the other side is like. We are in our "stuckedness" and we are fed by getting to be right about where we are. The more we talk about it, the more we can draw people into feeling sorry for us and not asking us to do things we are afraid of doing or things we simply just don't want to do.

Whatever is keeping us stuck in our comfort zone, even if it is an illness or debilitation, we use it as an excuse. The more we talk about it the more we believe it to be true, so we don't look for an alternative out of it. Even when an alternative is presented, we refuse to discuss it or accept that it could be an acceptable choice. Whatever IT is, IT is change, and change can be very difficult, especially when we are not ready to grow.

Soon after that experience, I learned I would be growing in an entirely different way! After two years of trying to get pregnant, I was told I would more than likely not be able to have children due to all the scar tissue from the abscesses. Miraculously, I did get pregnant. I remember the day I found out as if it were yesterday.

I stood up one day and almost passed out, and I had begun being very nauseated. I told my mother and she said, "It sounds like you're pregnant." Frustrated that she would even say that and having a bitter attitude about not being able to have children I so desperately wanted, I snapped that she knew that wasn't possible. I was stuck in my own beliefs and I didn't want to get excited about the possibility.

The girl that lived in our basement apartment worked at a urology clinic, so I let her take a urine specimen in to get tested. I was the "Tupperware Lady" and that day I had a morning demonstration party. Between burping lids and spinning salads I was hanging my head over the toilet. I don't know if it was the morning (actually all day) sickness, or the nerves of waiting for THE call that would be the biggest call of my life.

Suddenly the phone rang. I had told my hostess and guests what was up so they all gathered around. I remember standing in the kitchen of this strange house with a phone to my ear and hearing Linda say, "It's positive! You're pregnant!" I believe it was the happiest moment of my life.

The party was definitely over – I was crying so hard I couldn't even talk and I certainly didn't care if they knew how to burp those new lids! I just remember saying, "Here are the order forms and you better all order a lot because I am going to need the sales!" In that moment, I learned that anything is possible and you should never give up hope when there is something you want so desperately.

The next several months were grueling. I threw up 24/7. At five months pregnant and 5' 8" tall, I weighed only 109 pounds, and I would spend my second Christmas in the hospital. I clearly remember going to the emergency room on Christmas Eve and that handsome "Dr. Pat" was on call. I told him I was dehydrated and needed fluids and a shot of Phenergan. I knew the drill. I had been living it for five months.

He may have saved my life that day, or at least the life of my baby. He looked me straight in the eye and said in a rather irritated way, "Peggy, if you'd let me be the damn doctor and you be the patient we might find out what's going on with you! I AM admitting you to the hospital!"

I was dehydrated and I kept spiking a temperature, so they knew there was an infection somewhere. After a few days I had another fistula burst open. This time I was lucky – it opened to the outside instead of bursting inside.

I was in hysterics. All those memories of months in the hospital came flooding back. The local surgeon had come in my room and told me he felt certain they would be taking me to surgery and I would probably lose the baby. I remember yelling at him to get the hell out of my room. By then, my obstetrician had arrived from his office across the street. He came running into my room reassuring me no one was going to be doing surgery on me there, and he was calling Dr. Laws in Birmingham.

They finally figured out that somehow the pregnancy had triggered the internal pouch to start working which, in essence, was causing a continual blockage. I began using my catheter again and suddenly the nausea stopped and I was finally able to eat.

I gained about 30 pounds those last few months. On Easter Sunday at 11:00 p.m., I went into labor, and at 7:16 a.m., April 16, 1979, my little angel, Brooklyn, was born. At only five pounds, six ounces she was long, skinny and shriveled, but she was the most beautiful sight and the greatest gift God could have given me.

Two and a half months after she was born, I got the next greatest news of my life: I would be having another little bundle of joy in eight and a half months. My husband was in the hospital with meningitis when I got the news. I knew I needed to tell him before he came home from the hospital for fear he would have a heart attack. He had not weathered the first pregnancy well. I was ecstatic, my husband was in shock, and so was my doctor when I told him. My OBGYN wasn't ready to go through that again and suggested I shouldn't either. He was afraid for my health. I knew God would not have given me this second gift if I couldn't handle it, so I let the doctor know that I was having it so he better get ready. I remember him walking to his office muttering some four-letter words and shaking his head.

I knew what to expect and what to look for, and the next eight months went smoothly. I never even got sick. However, little Callie would be my stubborn one. She sat straight up in utero. She was not coming out, and if she was, it was her way – bottom first. Once again they were on the phone with Dr. Laws. They knew I had to have a cesarean section and they had no idea what they would be cutting into with my insides being totally rearranged. Dr. Laws, who was once on staff at our hospital in Anniston, came over from Birmingham to be there in case there was an emergency. Gotta love that man. On April 3, 1980, all went perfectly. Our little Callie was the most beautiful baby I had ever seen with her perfectly round head and just the right amount of hair.

I was given three miracles during that year. Two beautiful little girls and the internal pouch began working again out of the blue, so I was finally able to remove the bag and begin using my catheter to drain the pouch. It was great! However, I had learned to accept and live with wearing an external bag if that was what God had in store for me.

Unfortunately, as I had already begun to learn, life's ups often came with corresponding downs. My young husband was there with me through my struggles, but it took its toll on a young couple, and we struggled along for the next few years. I had grown so much during the ordeal and he had become stuck in a dark place – a comfort zone of his own. That comfort zone didn't include me and that became very uncomfortable. We couldn't survive it and we eventually went our separate ways; a decision that didn't come without guilt. I will be eternally grateful to him and his family for being there for me during that traumatic time in our lives. I just couldn't base forever on guilt.

Even though the odds were stacked against it, we were able

to have two beautiful daughters together. It was just another struggle in our relationship, but one well worth the fight.

Through my surgeries, my pregnancies, and even my new-found single life with babies, I learned so many lessons about life.

As I reflected on those lessons,

- I learned how important the right attitude is. especially when it comes to tough challenges in life.
- I learned about how my beliefs could really keep me stuck or help me move forward.
- I learned to be comfortable being uncomfortable.
- I learned about the power of choice when you are 10 feet from the edge.

I will share those lessons with you over the next several chapters, along with the steps you can take to help you through the tough times in life. I will share with you how you can learn to stretch your comfort zone one step at a time.

Are YOU ready to *stretch and grow?*

66 I am not my scars.
My scars are part of my beauty.
They are why I view life the way I
do today. Why I live life with

passion and purpose.

Why I understand the true value of life. 99

Chapter 5

Stretching
the
Comfort Zone

Having gone through the surgery ordeal, I had to develop a new comfort zone with my body. When I began dating after my divorce, I had to figure out when and with whom I would share my story. It was very personal to me and I had to decide how close I wanted to be to someone before sharing it. I was especially sensitive to this when it came time to discuss intimacy.

Most people in my situation might ask these questions. How do I explain to someone that I have a 21-inch-long by three-inch-wide scar from being left open to heal from the inside out? How do I explain that I wear this patch on my stomach because I don't go to the bathroom the way they do? What if I really started caring about someone and then they couldn't handle it? And worst of all – what if they rejected me because of it?

Although I admittedly had fleeting moments with those questions, I mostly chose to be upfront right from the beginning. I decided early on that if people couldn't accept me for who I was, with all my scars and body changes, they didn't belong in my life. I am not my scars. My scars are part of my beauty. They are why I view life the way I do today. Why I live life with passion and purpose. Why I understand the true value of life.

My comfort zone began stretching and growing in many directions. I was a single mom with one and two-year-old toddlers. The fear of raising them alone definitely expanded my comfort zone.

The maturity I had gained through my early ordeal led me

to relate better to someone much older than myself. I began dating again and met a gentleman named Gray, who was in the fashion business. I felt I had a tremendous amount in common with him.

I had attended or taught in a modeling school since I was 11 years old, and I had graduated from the Fashion Merchandising Institute after high school. Fashion was my passion, and the man I met owned the largest local department store downtown. He loved and accepted me with all my scars. He seemed to have a deep understanding of what I had experienced. I became more comfortable with the 24-year age difference, and over time we fell in love.

Our age difference didn't bother me, yet it seemed to bother a lot of other people in our small community. I had enough maturity and confidence in myself not to listen to the gossip. My mama would say, "If they're talking about you, they're just giving someone else a rest, so just ignore it." That was good advice. And hey, I was helping someone else by letting them talk about me – that was in my comfort zone!

I was 26 years old, and the opportunity arose for me to buy a modeling school 30 miles away. With Gray being in the fashion business, he thought it was a great idea, but told me he thought I needed a much shorter name for the door on my school. He explained that Peggy Hunter would look much better than Peggy Birchfield. And that was how he proposed to me!

We got married, and at the age of 26 I became a new business owner, starting a career of entrepreneurship.

I loved teaching personal development and motivating people to look at their lives differently. At times I taught up to 250 men, women, teens and children per year in my school. I had so much fun doing it. I discovered what Chaplain Bohannon meant by being able to add value to people's lives. This would become my life's passion and what I believe, was and is God's purpose in my life. I had CHOSEN to live for THIS purpose of making a difference in the lives of many.

Over the next 12 years I owned two schools and several satellite offices. I produced fashion shows for five apparel markets throughout the Southeast. That experience is a whole book of its own! I loved the path my career had taken me. I added value to the lives of many people, yet through the process, each of them added value to mine in a much greater way. Each school, each student and each project I took on stretched my comfort zone a little more.

My girls, Brooklyn and Callie, had grown up in my school. They had modeled since they were toddlers. Brooklyn had that gentle, mature attitude with an angelic look. Callie was the spunky, sassy one who knew how to command an audience from a very young age. After the second chance at life God had given me, they were the greatest gifts of my life.

In my marriage to Gray, I was gifted with being Stepmom to four other children from his previous marriages. Mark, the second oldest made our home his home away from college.

Although he was only six or seven years younger than I, he was my "baby boy" and I treated him like one of my kids. We still remain close after all these years.

At home, we were fortunate to have Irene, the woman who took care of the children, kept the house clean and prepared the food for our family. She was another member of our family and we helped each other through many trying times.

When the girls were about eight and nine years old, God blessed me with another beautiful gift.

Lisa, my best friend and partner at the time, and I were asked to coordinate and emcee one of the area high school beauty pageants. In our business, this was a regular occurrence, but this time would be very different.

We had awarded a full scholarship to our school to the winner of the pageant. The girl who won that night was so beautiful and deserving of the title of Miss Oxford. As it turned out, she was even more beautiful on the inside. Like me, she was a survivor. Not from health challenges but from life challenges. She had grown up with a mother who was plagued with addictions. In spite of the environment that would have swallowed up most kids and have them believe that was their destiny, she was a fighter. Tina knew she wanted more out of life, and modeling could be her way out.

God had something much bigger in store for us both. I was so impressed with her I hired her to teach at the school and to be a part-time nanny to my children. She became much more than that. She needed a family to love her and be there for her, and we were willing to be that family. We eventually adopted her as our own, and I have been blessed with being able to call her my daughter for more than 25 years now.

I watched her struggle to believe in herself. Then I watched her grow into a confident, beautiful woman, so talented and with so many gifts to share. We have been through some tough times together. She is my daughter and my friend and I couldn't love her more if she were my own blood.

During those same years, I began to realize, as I grew older and wiser, that I was stuck in another comfort zone. I realized that I was living under the control of my husband. I was not allowed to do the grocery shopping because I bought too much when I went. It made more sense to me that we saved money if I bought all the groceries for the month at one time, but my husband thought groceries should be bought weekly and somehow to him, $50 per week was less than $200 per month. It was also about him wanting us to eat his favorite cereal and his favorite ice cream – never about what we wanted. So I did what we do when we get stuck – I settled. I convinced myself that I didn't like to go grocery shopping anyway, so I was fine with it. There were other things I convinced myself of as well.

I almost convinced myself I should retire and sail off in to the wild blue yonder, but then a very wise friend and counselor reminded me that I was only 36 years old. He also told me I was the oldest 36-year-old woman he knew. I had begun to adapt to the stale routine of my 60-year-old husband's life, and I was drowning. I was dying a slow death and I had fought too hard to live to go there.

He was a good man, but we were killing each other. He was ready to retire yet I still had young children he felt responsible for, and he would have to work way beyond the years he had planned. The children "just being children" were difficult for him, and his expectations were hard on them. Sometimes you have to make choices in the best interest of all around you. My children were my life – they were my forever. We deserved to live in a growth environment, so I made a difficult choice.

I chose to step out of the marriage. Once again I would face the fear of being alone and making it on my own. We would go from living in the "big house on the hill" in the upscale neighborhood to living in the upstairs of the big house downtown where my school was located.

It wasn't long before I realized that in order to really grow; I needed to do something drastic.

"Your comfort zone

— not YOU — could be the one in control of everything you do in your life. Whatever place you are in, you likely created this space around what feels comfortable to you — it's your comfort zone. "

Chapter 6

Defining Moments

I remember the day and the moment very clearly. It was Easter Sunday of 1992. My husband and I had just separated and started divorce proceedings. Since we had lived in his family home, I had moved into the upstairs of the big antebellum home that my personal development and modeling school was located in.

On Easter Sunday, I took my girls for a picnic and some fresh air to one of my favorite spots, the highest point in Alabama – Cheaha State Park. Located just outside Anniston where we lived, the park is full of great trails where you can hike out to huge rock boulders and see for miles around.

We hiked down one trail to what is known as Pulpit Rock. From there you could see miles of natural beauty. It was a popular spot for climbing and rappelling off the 100-foot rock boulders. We walked up on to a large, flat rock and decided to settle into our picnic spot. As I placed my blanket and picnic items on the cool rock, the girls quickly and adventurously wandered across the rock to the edge to curiously look out into the valley. As they sat and dangled their feet freely over the edge, I felt the knot in my stomach forming.

I loved watching them enjoy their day – safely 10 feet from the edge. The breakup and move had been hard on them, and they deserved some fun time. Just watching them as they climbed the rocks and played so closely to the edge struck fear in me. My stomach was in knots and I kept cautioning them not to get too close and to be careful. I suddenly realized I was imposing my fear onto them. I knew it, but I just couldn't stop myself.

I wanted to pull them close into my comfort and safety zone. As young teens and pre-teens, they weren't listening very well, and now that I understand more clearly what was going on, I am glad they didn't. They kept teasing me about being a "scaredy cat" and kept coaxing me to move forward to see what they were seeing. And I did. Ever so slightly, scooting along on my bottom so I knew I was safely anchored to solid ground.

It seemed like such a simple day. A simple forgettable moment. But the truth is, it wasn't. It became a defining moment in my life. The fear I was feeling was not as much about falling off the edge of the rock; it represented my fear of being alone and wondering if I could do it once again. This time it would not be with two toddlers but with teenagers who embodied the eager and daring traits of once-small children. How would I manage it?

I had grown up in a small town and never left the comfort and safety of having my family close by. With the great trauma I had experienced early in life, my safety net had been made very clear. I went from my family home to being married, and I never lived all on my own. Even in the year and a half between my first husband and my second one, I had a friend living in the basement of my home. I was never really "alone" and making it on my own. But now I would be. After all, I was an adult in my late thirties. I was supposed to be able to do it. Of course I could bravely walk over to the edge of that rock and stand there. But I couldn't. It was out of my comfort zone, the place where I felt safe.

As I sat and watched the kids climb the rocks and watched the people across the way squealing with joy as they rappelled down that 100-foot rock cliff, I wondered. I wondered to myself if I would ever be able to walk to the edge by myself. Would I ever be able to survive on my own with teenage children? Where was my life headed? What would change?

Just at that moment, a tall, slender guy walked up beside me. I was sitting 10 feet back from the edge. Ten feet from freedom of fear, anxiety and loss of control. He plunked down a bag full of ropes, straps and rappelling gear. I looked up at him and asked, "Is that mountain climbing gear?" He replied that it was for rock rappelling.

At that moment I boldly said something I couldn't believe was coming out of my mouth.

I exclaimed, "I WANT TO DO THAT!"

Did those words REALLY just come out of my mouth? Deep inside I was screaming, "WAIT, let me rewind and take that back!"

He calmly said, "I have extra gear if you want to come along." At that moment, fear and panic set in and I was suddenly feeling the same loss of control I felt as my marriage went over the edge.

I guess he could see the dread in my eyes as well as the clinch in my body. My butt glued to the rock, my legs pressed flat against the solid surface, and my hands desperately trying to grip it as tightly as possible! Every part of my body was anchored to that rock. Ten feet from the edge and cemented to my comfort zone. Of course it didn't help that my kids had now become involved actively in the conversation, shouting, "We want to do it! She's a scaredy cat ... she won't do it! Take us!"

He calmly looked down into my eyes and said "I am an instructor and I would be happy to teach you how. I will be right by your side to make sure you are safe." He somehow knew what I needed to hear. At that moment, he reached down with his hand and held it out to help me up. I stared at his hand for what seemed like eternity, then I reached up and clasped on tight as I slowly unglued myself from the rock.

DEFINING *Moment*

In that moment I chose to step out of the safety of my comfort zone and to stretch and grow. I had NO idea how that one short moment, that one bold decision, would affect the rest of my life.

DEFINING the *Comfort Zone*

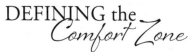

What is it we mean by "comfort zone"? Well, in looking at the freedictionary.com site, it defines it as "a situation or position in which a person feels secure, comfortable, or in control. So let's break that down further and see how each of the key words are defined:

SITUATION = the combination of circumstances at any given moment; or a way in which something is positioned; or a position or status with regard to conditions or circumstances.

SECURE = Free from danger, risk, fear, anxiety or doubt; not likely to fail.

Comfortable = Free from stress or anxiety; physical comfort; feelings of ease or security; to provide financial security.

IN *Control* = to exercise authoritative or dominating influence over; authority or ability to manage or direct.

So, what it really means is that at any given moment we are aware of our surroundings so we feel free from risk, anxiety, stress or danger. By knowing we are able to exercise authority and control over any given situation, we have the ability to manage our circumstances. It is our safe place.

Think about it. What is your "safe place" with your mate, your job, your social life, and even with your play time? Your comfort zone – not YOU – could be the one in control of everything you do in your life. In your relationships, your comfort zone controls how close you get, how many times you go out, what house you live in, how far you take your intimacy. In your job, your comfort zone could be sitting behind a desk assisting others being the one who leads a team, or the one who loves to be out selling to clients. In your social life, you could be completely comfortable staying home all to yourself or out socializing and loving to be the life of the party. And your play time comfort zone could be 10 feet back on that rock or out parasailing, skydiving and always looking for the next thrill. Whatever place you are in, you likely created this space around what feels comfortable to you – it's your comfort zone.

IS THERE DANGER in the *Comfort Zone?*

YES, but what's wrong with staying safely in your comfort zone? Here's the real danger: When you settle into a comfort zone and refuse to step outside that boundary, you are basically saying THIS IS IT! This is all I will EVER be in this situation for the rest of my life.

Here is what you need to always remember: As a once dear friend of mine said, "If you don't stay green and growing, you will ripen and rot!" Do you want to ripen and rot? If not, then boldly step outside your comfort zone!

Your comfort zone really is just about habits you have created in your life that happen without any thought. Remember when you were finally old enough to learn to drive a car? You had dreams and visions of one day driving that car by yourself. Because you would turn driving age before all your friends, you would be the cool kid who could drive everyone around to the hangout places. You would not have to be dependent on your parents to take you anywhere ever again. You couldn't wait for the vision you could clearly see becoming a reality.

The big day came for you to drive the car for the first time. You were so excited about getting behind that wheel, but when you did, you soon developed white knuckle syndrome. Gripping the wheel so tight and feeling so out of control and riddled with anxiety. You barely mashed the gas pedal, and when you tried to mash it just a little harder, you jerked that car right down the asphalt. The more you practiced, the more comfortable you became. Soon you were confidently hopping in that car and it was smooth sailing! (In the parking lot of the church, of course.) Did you really think you would start out on the road with other people?

Then you became comfortable driving around the parking lot. Heck, you could even turn all the corners sharply between the lines in that big parking lot, and you could even pull right into the parking space. Of course, there's no need to mention there were no other cars in that lot during the middle of the weekday. Then one day, it was time for the next step, crossing the street where other cars may actually be in motion, to get yourself to the church parking lot across the way. OH NO!!! I'm not ready! I have to cross a REAL street! So, the brakes come on and you wait for the perfect moment, looking both ways a dozen times, then WHAM! You gun it across that street, bottoming out as you fly to the next parking lot. You slam on the brakes with your heart pounding and you look around. Knowing it was not a smooth crossing, you still felt the success of doing it and you shout out, "I did it! I did it!" It did not matter that you scared your poor mother to death. You did it! Yes, I know this story so well because I lived it with three girls.

And then one day it's time to stretch again. To get outside that comfort zone of the church parking lot. You are scared, but you do it because you know you have a goal. You can feel what it feels like to be the cool kid who can drive everyone around. Oh, you want that feeling so badly. You know the only way to get that feeling is to be able to drive by yourself one day. So you stretch. You are not only driving, but being driven. Something outside of you is now propelling you forward. Your heart pounds as you see that first car coming past and you wonder if you can do it. Will I hit him? Am I over far enough? Can I do this? And then suddenly the next thing you know, you are not only past that car but you have now passed three more. You feel the confidence of that stretch. You have a new comfort zone.

Then the day comes when dad says, "Let's go out onto the highway and really floor this thing!" Once again you experience all the emotions around stepping out of something that is so comfortable, so safe, to go into the unknown. You experience something bigger than you had moments ago. Your growth begins outside the comfort zone. It wasn't really so bad, was it? Now, you are driving down the road, talking on the phone, brushing your hair, and eating your sandwich. You need both hands to do that so you use your knee to steer the wheel. Driving is now such a habit you don't even think about it. Sometimes you even drive a few miles before realizing how far you have gone because you are simply doing what is subconsciously normal and comfortable.

This is what happens in life. We have a tendency to get extremely comfortable just doing what comes naturally, and we don't even realize how stuck we are. How much life has passed by … how many opportunities have we missed because we sold out to our comfort zone. We lose sight of the feeling of that goal of being the cool kid who can drive everyone else around, or we quit setting goals all together. Our relationships become routine, our jobs become mundane, and our existence becomes repetitive. And we stay there – ripening and rotting 10 feet from the edge.

66 *There are times in life*
where we just have to

take a chance

and just do it.
Whatever IT is. 99

FEAR =
False **E**vidence **A**ppearing **R**eal

Chapter 7

Fear is Temporary.
Regret is Forever.

When I made the decision to trust a stranger to safely guide me through my first rappelling experience, I was taking a big step outside my comfort zone. A BIG step! We moved to a new location better for rappelling. The girls were really excited that I was going to do it, and they were in a bit of a state of disbelief. My new friend, the rappelling instructor, was coaching me through how to put all the safety harnesses on, and then I watched as he anchored the end of the rope to a tree a few feet back from the edge.

He carefully explained to me that he would rappel down first and wait at the bottom for my cue. Once I was ready, he would belay the rope, securing me (the climber) while I made my descent down the 100-foot rock face. All I needed to do was to hold on to the rope, turn my back to the cliff and lay back into thin air with my body parallel to the ground and my feet planted on the rocks. I thought, "YOU WANT ME TO DO WHAT? Lay out in thin air trusting the rope is firmly tied and won't come loose? You are kidding me, right?"

This was the point I wanted to run safely back to my comfort zone 10 feet from the edge and plaster myself against that rock! He just kept reassuring me by saying, "You will be OK. I will be down at the bottom waiting for you and I won't let you fall!" With hesitation, I let him walk me over to the edge, showing me how the harness and the rope "had me locked in safely." Then he said something very profound. He said, "You will not fail at this. You are safe." And off he went, to the bottom – 100 feet down!

After he got down there, he shouted up to me and told me to go ahead, he had the rope. I stood back from that ledge, contemplating what was about to happen. It was the first of many defining moments that day. My heart was racing. Flashes of my life began running through my head. I was remembering the first time I did a front handspring; the first time I drove a car; the first day I saw the toilet filled with blood; the day they took me to surgery for the first time, then the second and then the third. I was remembering the fight for my life and the time they told me my first born might have to be taken at just five months into the pregnancy. I remembered the feeling of opening my first business; standing on the stage for the first time to speak to a large audience; and as my next thought switched to moving out on my own with three teens I realized I was recalling the most fearful moments in my life. And now rappelling ranked right up there at the top with the other most fearful moments.

So many times before I had ventured outside of my comfort zone and stepped over the edge. Each time I had survived. Why was I so paralyzed now? And then I realized I had been standing on that ledge for almost 30 minutes contemplating all of my biggest fears. My senses were so numbed I couldn't even hear the words the nice instructor below was patiently saying to me. I was stuck and frozen in fear.

Out of nowhere it seemed, a really good looking guy walked up to me. He was tall, a little rugged, with sandy blonde hair and big blues eyes that sparkled. Evidently he had been watching me stand there in a place he had been before. He looked at me and said, "You're probably scared to death about now, huh?" I nodded at him with tears in my eyes. In a consoling way, he reassured me I would be all right and that he would stand there with me. I told him that I wanted so badly to do this, but I couldn't move past the fear.

He could see the fear on my face, and like the angel in my hospital room, he looked at me and said, "You have a choice. You don't have to go over that edge. There are no HAVE to's in life. There are only GET to's. I will undo your gear and you can walk away never having faced your fear, but I can promise, you will live with regret. What will it be?"

I remember looking deep in his blue eyes – it was almost as if I was looking into my own soul. A calm came over me. I said, "NO, I HAVE to. Correction – I GET to do this!"

That's when he said something that would stay with me forever. My defining moment number two in this day. He simply said, "FEAR is False Evidence Appearing Real. It keeps us stuck in our comfort zone way too often."

I told him I didn't want to be stuck in my comfort zone. That I had to get out of it to survive what I was going through. As I was saying that he was gently turning me around with my back to the ledge and backing me up closer. At this time I was standing with my heels right at the edge of that rock cliff. He just calmly said, "Look in my eyes. Don't look at anything else." He gently placed his hands on my arms and said, "I've got you. Just start slowly leaning back. The rope is tight and you won't fall."

The next thing I knew I was hanging parallel to the ground. He let me stay there a little bit while he continued talking. He was telling me that there are times in life where we just have to take a chance and just do it. Whatever "it" was to me. Then he calmly said, "Just bend your knees slightly and push off with your feet and take a short hop on the rock. Look at you! You're doing great! You are rappelling!"

My kids were cheering me on, the instructor was cheering me on and my confidence grew. Suddenly I realized I was about 10 feet down. I was looking in his eyes still and tears were flowing from mine. All of the sudden I felt this exhilarating feeling.

I AM DOING THIS!

I CAN DO THIS!

I AM ON MY OWN AND I AM EXCITED!

I looked back toward the ground and shouted "I'M COMING DOWN!" Then I looked back up at the angel up top and shouted, "I WOULD MARRY YOU IF YOU WEREN'T ALREADY MARRIED! THANK YOU! THANK YOU! YES! I CAN DO THIS!"

I pushed out and hopped a little further down the rock, then again and again until I felt the instructor reach up for me. We all celebrated and laughed about how long it had taken me to take that first step over the edge. THEY laughed even harder when I realized I now had to climb back up that rock face to get out of there!

That day, two strangers helped me break through the fear barrier. Intellectually, I knew I was going to be safe. I knew there were dozens of others out on those rocks having a great time rappelling and they were all safe. But I let fear take over. I let the false evidence of my beliefs appear real to me. In some way, I knew if I could go down that 100-foot rock cliff, I could make it on my own with my teenage girls and my business. I knew if I could do that, I could do ANYTHING. And that scared me, too. IF I did this, then I would have no excuse to not succeed. I could do it, all on my own, knowing that my family would always be there belaying my rope if I really needed them to.

How many times have you been so afraid of failing you sold out on yourself about something you really wanted in life? And for what? So you could sit back and play the regret game? Some of us even convince ourselves we didn't really want that anyway, like it was just a fleeting thought.

I often have coaching clients who come to me because they are stuck and they just don't understand why they can't move forward. In most of the cases when we drill down through the coaching process, they discover there is one of two things holding them back: fear or self-limiting beliefs. And in most cases, our fears COME from our self-limiting beliefs.

What's most important? You must know your purpose and connect with your passion in order to stay in action and push through fear. What are you afraid of? What in your life requires ACTION? Living a life based on fear is a hard way to live. When you choose to step out and break through and take action ANYWAY, it is the most liberating experience ever!

I was so excited after I successfully made it to the bottom of the rappelling adventure. Then I suddenly realized I had to climb back up the rock to go home. Oh my! With my newly stretched comfort zone, it was not as scary as it was taking that first step over the ledge and then going down the cliff. That is the beauty of getting unstuck and doing whatever it is that you may be afraid of doing.

UNDERSTANDING *Fear*

The truth is our fears don't really exist. We create the fears and live inside of them. Fear can just be thoughts that make your brain react in a way that signals your body to go into fight or flight mode. Let's take a look at what happens:

- THOUGHTS create FEAR

- The MIND sends a signal to the BRAIN

- The BRAIN says "OH NO! We're in danger!
  I must send a signal to the BODY!"

- The BODY says "CODE RED! CODE RED!
  Prepare for DANGER!"

- The BODY then goes into FIGHT OR FLIGHT
  mode and your blood pressure rises, you become
  tense in the neck, your stomach churns and
  you become short of breath.

SO WHAT DO YOU DO?

Breathe. Yes, breathe. Take a deep breath. When you do this, the body then says "Wow, we must not be running because we're taking too long to breathe, so I'll send a signal back to the brain that we must not be in danger." Then the brain says, "Oh, I'll tell the mind not to worry or be afraid." And suddenly you don't feel that strong sense of fear any longer. So just take a deep breath and do it anyway!

An exercise you can do to help you relax and push through is to flex your entire body. Start with your fists and move up your arms to your head, then down your torso to your feet, flexing every part of your body and then relaxing it. Alternate between breathing normally and breathing slowly and deeply into the lungs. If you do this for three minutes before you do something which is causing you fear such as giving a speech, confronting an employee, (or even stepping off a 100-foot cliff with a rope tied around you), what you will experience is a resetting of the nervous system. As a result, you'll calm your state of mind. By resetting the physiology, you feel more relaxed.

To help on a more long term basis, eliminate caffeine, sugar, and other stimulants – these actually fuel the fight-or-flight response.

You should also avoid people who reinforce your fear. We call these biological irritants. Yes, there are actually people out there who get their satisfaction by instilling fear in others. They might just be family members or so called friends. Stick close to emotional nurturers and those who help you feel better about yourself. Stay away from violent newscasts, movies that illicit fear, arguments, or other stress inducers. Many adults are afraid of flying because they watched one too many airplane crash movies or they won't go in the ocean or water they can't see the bottom of because they watched too many creature movies. These are images that become very real in our brains and help to keep us stuck, fearful and uncomfortable, preventing us from doing things we might really want to do.

Now let's also discuss the fact that some fear is very real and very necessary. When you are in a state of real danger, such as someone physically trying to harm you or in emergency situations, don't take time to do the deep breathing thing. Just run like hell! You don't want your body to go into calm, safe mode; you want it to stay in fight or flight mode.

You might find you are one of those people who remain very calm when there is an emergency, but when it is all over the fear sets in and you feel the panic symptoms of fear.

I remember the day I was sitting in a Wendy's restaurant having a leisurely lunch with a friend from New York who was down doing some training in my school. All the sudden a man just fell out of his chair and onto the floor. It was obvious he was struggling to breathe, and then he quit breathing. I followed my instinct to get up and help. It seemed there were only two of us in the restaurant that day who knew CPR, myself and the FedEx guy. We immediately began loosening his clothes. In fact, I realized in the panic of the moment I had actually unbuckled and unzipped his pants as well!

After administering CPR, he began breathing again, but just barely, so we continued until the ambulance arrived. After it was all over, I had my panic moment where I broke down and felt the fear. I had to do some serious deep breathing.

About a month later, a woman walked into my school and sat quietly on the chair in front of my desk. I asked if I could help her and she simply said, "The man in Wendy's was my husband. I just wanted to come by and say thank you for what you did. That's all, just thank you." Unfortunately he did not survive as he had suffered a massive heart attack. She stood up and gave me a hug and left. I never even knew her name. After she left, I thought about all the people in that restaurant who just sat there in fear, not knowing what to do or too afraid to do anything. My own friend had just continued eating his lunch. Fear can be paralyzing if you give into it or if you let it consume you.

Psychoanalyst Dr. Alexander Lowen believed fear could be traced to the fear of life. In his book *Fear of Life*, he said, "Fear of life can be seen in the way we keep busy so as not to feel, keep running so as not to face ourselves, or get high on liquor or drugs so as not to sense our being. Because we are afraid of life, we seek to control or master it. We believe it is bad or dangerous to be carried away by our emotions. We admire the person who is cool, who acts without feeling. The modern individual is committed to being successful, not to being a person. He belongs rightly to the 'action generation' whose motto is do more but feel less."

Have you ever found yourself so fearful of life you become paralyzed, or you keep yourself so busy you don't have to feel? I am sure most of us have done that at some point. The problem comes when you become stuck in that fear. So stuck you can't move forward and you run back to that point 10 feet away from the edge, safely in your comfort zone.

What are you fearful of? What are you not doing because you are too afraid?

Here's an exercise to help you overcome the fear and take action:

1 Ask yourself the question, "What am I not doing because I am too afraid?" Then answer it on paper. Sit down and write out all the things you have not done because you were afraid to step out of your comfort zone.

2 Beside each, rank them on a scale of one to 10 (with one being the lowest) by how committed you are to breaking through your comfort zone for that item.

3 Then rank them in order by how much each has affected your life, held you back, or kept you from moving forward.

4 Now pick the top three and write out, in detail, what you will do to take action toward eliminating them from the list. For example, if you ranked yourself a five on your commitment level, then write out the steps that would get you to a commitment

level of six. You only want to move up one step at a time, so when you get to a six, decide what it will take to get to a seven.

5 After you have eliminated those three fears or holdbacks, write down the next three most important ones and repeat the action all over again.

Let's say you really have wanted to talk to your boss about a raise, and that is the number one thing on your list you want to resolve. Your commitment level is at a four because you have a lot of fear about doing this. So what will it take to get to a five? Maybe you need to find someone to coach you through why you are so afraid so a five step would be searching for an accessible coach. You complete that, so to get to a six you actually make an appointment with two or three of them for a consultation to help you discover the right coach for you. To get to a seven, you make a commitment to work with the coach you have chosen. To get to an eight, you do the work to breakthrough what is holding you back. To get to a nine, you make an appointment with your boss. At a 10, you are sitting in front of your boss having a well-thought-out discussion about why you deserve a raise.

It is great if you get the raise, but even if you don't, you have still won the battle between you and your comfort zone. As you do this, you will begin to grow forward slowly and intentionally. You will begin to stretch your comfort zone and live on the outer edge of fear. You learn how to master overcoming fear, how to begin to feel comfortable feeling uncomfortable. If you don't prioritize overcoming fear, it will overcome you.

“ *Often times when we get stuck in our*

comfort zone,

we allow OTHERS to direct our lives.
Even when we know it is wrong. We just give the
power over to them willingly as if we're saying,
'You can run my life better than I can. **”**

Chapter 8

Crazy
Stupid
Choices

Life. It's just that simple. It really is. Until you make stupid choices! That's right. The bottom line is, WE complicate life by the choices we make. Think about it, how many really dumb choices have you made in your life? I'm not talking about the big ones; I'm talking about all those little ones that add up.

Have you ever had three cups of coffee then hopped in the car for a two-plus hour commute? Now you are fully aware that coffee is going to go straight through you and you know you will be doing the "car seat shuffle" as I call it. Then you decide to complicate things. You know the point will come when you will have to find a place to stop along the way. You pass the first exit because you thought you would find a better place right up the road, then realize there are no more exits nearby! So you are then contemplating pulling off the side of the road! By this time, your teeth are floating and you just know you're not going to make it. Been there, done that, got the T-shirt. Stupid little choices that complicate our lives.

I am a big proponent of setting goals. If they are good goals, they will stretch us beyond our comfort zone. I teach a class on Purpose, Vision and Goals and the importance of designing your life rather than having someone else design it for you. Often times when we get stuck in our comfort zone, we allow OTHERS to direct our lives. Even when we know it is wrong. We just give the power over to them willingly as if we're saying, "You can run my life better than I can." How does that work for you? Not very well if you really want to achieve your goals and dreams.

I have always been a goal-setter, and when I set a goal, I usually achieve it. Even when I was a kid I did that. I remember this one weekend in June when I was 18 years old. We had just graduated high school, and one of my best friends was getting married on Saturday night. I was one of her bridesmaids.

The Miss Talladega 500 pageant was the same night as the wedding and I really wanted to enter it because you got two grandstand tickets to the race for being a contestant. We lived just 20 miles or so from the raceway so it was always fun to go. Actually, what I would do is sell the two high-priced tickets and buy several infield tickets for all my friends.

I had set my goal to get those grandstand tickets, and I had it figured out pretty well, I thought. The judge's interview was on Saturday at 1:00 p.m., so I would have plenty of time to go there and get back for the wedding at five. I knew I could slip out of the reception between 6:30 to 7:00 and make the 30-minute drive to Talladega for the pageant, which started at eight. I had a friend who was going to drive me so I could change gowns on the way over. Good plan, win-win-right? Until I complicated it.

The night before the wedding we had a bachelorette party at the local motel everyone was staying in, and there was alcohol involved. They were going to play a game. I was not much of a drinker so I didn't fully understand the impact of playing a shot game with vodka. I must have lost a lot of the rounds. The last thing I remembered was being pushed in the pool and landing on my head in the shallow end.

The next morning, as I thought I was awakening out of a restful night, I was having this really weird dream. In my dream I was lying in the bathtub with the shower running on me and my mother was yelling, "Where are your teeth?" You see, I was genetically missing the two teeth on either side of my two front teeth, and I wore a partial with two artificial teeth attached to it. The partial was made of plastic. It fit up in the roof of my mouth and the teeth looked quite natural.

As I began to move around a bit and waken further, I realized I was lying on a rubber mattress pad in my daddy's robe. Was this part of my dream still? Oh, no – this was the real thing! As I sat up in the bed and looked around, things were different. My covers were replaced with an old blanket, and there was a trash can by my bed. I got up and went into the bathroom, still trying to wake up and figure out what had happened, when suddenly my mother walked into the room. Well, I can tell you, the wrath of my mother could be a big one, and when I looked at her face I saw it coming.

I looked up and said, "What happened?" And she didn't waste any time telling me! "You were disgustingly drunk! We heard you come in, and then we thought we heard footsteps leave, and then we heard you hiccupping loudly and then just laughing hysterically in the bed. Then we heard something else. We got up to see what was going on, and you were lying there throwing up all over yourself and the bed. We finally got you out of bed and into the shower. That's when we realized your daddy had flushed your teeth down the toilet with everything else you threw up! What on earth did you think you were doing? How foolish could you be?" And it went on and on. I definitely complicated my life and everyone else's that day!

It wasn't long after I got up and started moving around that I had my head back in the toilet again. I was SO sick, and all I could think was how on earth am I going to go to Talladega for that judges interview as sick as I was. Oh – and just to make matters worse, I had NO TEETH! Well Mama began feeding me chicken noodle soup, because in the south, it's good for everything, and Daddy started feeding me pink Pepto-Bismol to try to settle my stomach. I was in a panic because I had a beauty pageant AND a wedding to be in and I was missing two of my front teeth!

I suddenly remembered I had an old partial I had saved for some reason. (Turns out this was the reason!) I was really upset because it didn't really fit, but all Mother and Daddy were worried about was what they would tell the dentist about why I had to have a new partial. You see, he and his wife were some of their closest friends, and they were very religious. How humiliated they would be to have to tell him the truth that their daughter, his girls' close friend, had done something so unacceptable. Keep in mind, I grew up in a household where I never saw my parents take a drink until I was almost an adult.

All I know is, on the way to Talladega for the judges' interview I left a trail of pink noodles all along the roadside! But that wasn't the worst of it. I am just here to tell you, you cannot talk very well with a partial that doesn't fit your mouth. Every time I went to talk, my teeth would slip down. This talkative girl was not doing a lot of talking when the judges asked their questions! Are you kidding me? I couldn't even smile without my teeth falling down. It was not a good day. Life could have been so simple, but I complicated it through stupidity. However, I had a goal in mind! I was getting those tickets!

We rushed back to Anniston after that horrible experience, and I changed into my bridesmaid's dress in the car on the way back. During the wedding, I damn near passed out as I stood there praying they would hurry up and say their vows and be done. I did not feel good because I could not keep anything down all day and was quite dehydrated. This day and time, I would swear it was alcohol poisoning or maybe I had a concussion from the fall in the pool. Surely I could not be this sick from drinking a little alcohol! (Well, maybe it was a lot of alcohol!)

When that wedding was over, I jumped back in the car and I pushed through because I had a goal. I was getting those grandstand tickets to the Talladega 500 Race. At this point it wasn't about winning a pageant. I knew they were not going to give the title to a girl who couldn't talk because her teeth kept falling out. But I put on my evening gown, mustered up the last bit of strength I had and I walked down that runway with a simple closed-mouth smile, and finally it was over. I had my tickets. I had achieved my goal. And I had learned a very valuable lesson. Several actually. They were:

1 Never play a shot game again with alcohol.

2 Sometimes you can get so far out of your comfort zone it's

dangerous. (God was with me that night – the outcome could have been far worse.)

3 You can achieve any goal you want when you really feel the vision in your heart. It doesn't matter what challenges are there, you will find a way.

Finally Don't complicate life any more than you have to.

JUST KEEP IT SIMPLE.

Talking about the choices we make every day. How many of you have reached over and turned off the alarm at 6:00 a.m. only to say to yourself, "I'll just lie here five more minutes." Then, yep! You wake up at 7:30 and you have a really important meeting you're in charge of at 8:00 and it's across town. Not a smart choice.

This list of stupid choice examples can go on and on and on. They add up! We won't even talk about the big ones like getting married to my high school sweetheart at 19. You make a lot of bad choices at that age in life. You think you know it all, but of course, you don't. But I will say, in my case, he gave me two of the most incredible blessings in my life, my two amazing daughters who brought me so much joy. Until they became teenagers and started making their own stupid choices! Just kidding – even with all the crazy choices they made, my daughters have been the pure joy and happiness in my life. Especially with the seven (at the time of this writing) beautiful grandchildren they have brought into my life. I wouldn't trade a day of all the blessings I have as a result of the two I birthed, the one I adopted and the two I was gifted with my forever husband.

You see, even those crazy stupid choices can turn out to be the greatest gifts. Sometimes it's through the lessons you learn, sometimes it's through the beauty that comes as a result of it. The difference is whether or not you grow from it. If you learned something and grew from it in the process, then it may have been a stupid choice worth making.

It's the attitude you have in life about the choices you make that determines if you are growing and getting the results you want. I can tell you a lot about attitudes, and I think I will!

*66 Some believe our attitude can be genetic.
I believe it is also*

who we have learned to be

*based on our beliefs, our values and the
way we see ourselves at that moment. 99*

Chapter 9

A = *Attitude*

In the A, B, C's of life, A = Attitude. When you think of attitude, what do you think of? Attitudes can be good or bad, and they can sometimes be indifferent. Interestingly enough, most people immediately think of the person they know who has a bad attitude. What does that say about us?

Let me ask you another question. Where do attitudes come from? Here is the answer I like best: Everything begins with thoughts and feelings about where we are at any specific moment in life. These thoughts and feelings manifest into attitudes that either serve us well or destroy us.

After going through such a life-altering illness early in my life, I got to CHOOSE what my attitude would be about a lot of different things. The attitude I would choose would either destroy me or propel me forward. In my senior year of high school I had to give up cheerleading, something I loved so much. Yet, I had lost so much weight due to my illness, I was the perfect size for modeling. That became my new passion and it became my career in my early years.

Someone asked me once: What is the primary cause of your results? HMMMMM ... that's a deep one! Because of everything I had been through, I had to search my heart to get to the answer to that question. I thought about all the times I had been most successful in business and the happiest and most content in life. I thought about all the times life seemed to flow and the times I struggled the most. I looked at the times I was the happiest and the times I was at my lowest. The times I had bounced back in life, like after my surgeries. Or after my second divorce when I made the decision to move to Florida. Within a month of making that decision, I had packed up my life and my kids, closed the business I had owned for 12 years, left everything behind I had known for the first 37 years of my life and moved to a strange place. I had no idea what I was going to do or how I was going to do it. I just knew I had to do something to move my life forward in a big way.

I looked at how I had survived that horrible nightmare of six months in the hospital at such a young, fragile age. I knew the primary cause of the results in my life. I knew it was the fact that I had chosen to have a positive attitude in the face of all that challenged me. But where did that come from? Some believe our attitude can be genetic. I believe it is also who we have learned to be based on our beliefs, our values and the way we see ourselves in that moment.

The scary thing is our attitude controls every aspect of our lives. What does your attitude say about you? When something bad happens, do you look for the lessons in it and find the positive or do you immediately go to a place of doom and gloom? Or worse yet, blame? Often times because our beliefs about ourselves, I call them the "bees." You know – the ones that sit on your shoulder and buzz in your ear. "THEY chose that restaurant and THEY know I don't like the food there." (Granted you had a voice in the decision but chose not to use it.) Or "THEY don't care what my opinion is … blah, blah, blah." Whatever your "bees" may be, the outcome is still the same.

You get frustrated, angry and go into the "woe is me" mode.

STOP! What if they forgot you didn't like the food there? What if one of the group members really wanted to go there because it was her mom's favorite place and she had lost her mom this time a year ago? She may not have shared that. What if this? What if that? You get the picture. It doesn't always have to be about YOU.

I remember when I was in the hospital and after four months of not eating and not moving out of the bed, I had to learn to walk again due to muscle atrophy. I was feeling really sorry for myself because it was a struggle. I would tell them "I'm not up to going today." One day they said, "We want you to meet someone. He will be going with you to physical therapy. He is a little younger than you but he is learning to walk again also." I was intrigued.

The next day we stopped on the way to pick up another patient. When they brought him out in his wheelchair, I was confused. How on earth was he going to learn to walk? He had no legs and no arms, or at least very little of them. His legs were formed to just above his knees. One arm came to just above the elbow and one formed into one finger just below the elbow. WOW! And here I was feeling sorry for myself and my situation! Mine was at least temporary. This young man was 14 years old and he was born this way. He was going to physical therapy because they had made new legs for him and he was going to learn to walk on them.

Needless to say, I was inspired to go to physical therapy each day. Each day I would watch him hop out of his wheelchair and onto the mat. Then he would put the legs on they had made for him and attempt to walk. At first it was a challenge for him, but he never gave up, and soon he got the hang of it. While I watched him, I too was getting out of my wheelchair and building up my muscles to walk again.

For food at the time? All I could do was suck on hard candy and drink liquids. I would take him individually wrapped hard candy each day and I would watch in amazement how he was able to open the wrapper. And I watched in awe at how positive his attitude was. It inspired me to change mine on those hard days. I don't remember the boy's name but I do remember the visual and the impact it had on my life. I understood the power of a positive attitude, and that it was a choice we could make and should make each day of our life.

I was called to remember this story again recently, when I had the good fortune to witness another amazing man in action: Nick Vujicic of the Life Without Limbs Organization. Look him up online. Buy his book and movie. He travels around the world inspiring people in a huge way. Once you see Nick in action and see him speak, you really get the opportunity to check your attitude. Here is this man whose body is a torso with a head and one little foot with two toes where his right leg should be. He may not have arms and legs, but he has a heart as big as the world. He lives his life with NO ARMS – NO LEGS – NO LIMITS. He types 43 words per minute with those two little toes! Makes you kind of ask yourself what your own excuses are, doesn't it?

As a speaker, I sometimes wonder how I am going to get through a 90-minute or two-hour speaking engagement. I watched him stand on that table on stage and work it from side to side with an energy and enthusiasm that would motivate anyone to action. I will never complain again that my feet hurt or that I am tired of standing!

Born in Melbourne, Australia, Nick refused to allow his physical condition to limit his lifestyle. There was a time when he was very young that he questioned the purpose of life, or if he even had a purpose. According to Nick, the victory over his struggles, as well as his strength and passion for life today, can be credited to his faith in God, his family, friends and the many people along the journey who have inspired him to carry on. He is a true testament to the power of a positive attitude, and the power of getting up each day and carrying on in the face of challenges. He is an inspiration to all who encounter him. Look him up on YouTube the next time you are having a "bad attitude" day.

We all go through challenging times in life. It's the attitude we CHOOSE with the challenge that makes or breaks us. When I was sick with the debilitating ulcerative colitis, someone once told me something that always stuck with me. They said, "You can't change the disease you have and the situation it has created. All you can change is your attitude about it." Your attitude is your choice and has nothing to do with anything or anyone else.

I used to tell my students, when you wake up in the morning, look in the mirror and say, "It's a GREAT day and I am a beautiful person!" Say it with passion and conviction. Say it daily until you believe it and then have an attitude of gratitude for the beautiful person you are and for the beautiful day before you.

66 *What have you missed out*
on in life because of the

'bee-liefs' you have created

about yourself based on
someone else's opinion? **99**

Chapter 10

B = Bee-liefs...
$Bzzzz$

Your beliefs ... the "bees" on your shoulder.

What are they *buzzing* in your ear?

- You can't do that, you're not smart enough!
- Why would you think he/she would give you the time of day?
- You're not worthy of having that.
- You're too short/tall – fat/skinny – young/old – ugly/pretty – to do THAT!
- Why would you think you're smart enough for THAT?
- You didn't go to college or you didn't finish high school.
- You're not good enough for him/her.
- You'll never be anything!
- They don't want to hear what you have to say!
- You talk too much!
- You're too stupid!
- You need to stand in the corner and hum because your voice is not made for singing.
- You're too shy – you've always been the shy one.
- You're just a dreamer – get your head out of the clouds!
- You don't come from the right side of the tracks!

And on, and on like a broken record these words play in your head. What are your "bees" and how long will you choose to let them keep controlling your life?

Often our "bees" – our beliefs about ourselves – are imparted on us by someone else. Sometimes it is the ones who are supposed to love us the most who bestow these buzzing creatures on our shoulders and in our hearts and minds.

The tough thing is, in that one instance when a statement is made or an action happens, it changes our lives forever. Sometimes it happens because of what other kids say about us in school. Sometimes it is what a family member says and sometimes it is what they say because in their mind they are trying to help you or make you feel better.

It could be as simple as not getting invited to a party or a dance. At that moment we formulate a belief about ourselves that stays with us the rest of our lives. It's really sad how this happens. Let me share a story of a wonderful woman I met.

She was a young college student in a small private school that only had three sororities. She had always been a bright, bubbly girl and was quite beautiful. She waited until her second year of college to go out for rush week because she wanted to get that first year under her belt and she wanted to make sure she would make the right choice when it came to choosing a sorority.

The big week finally came – Sorority Rush Week. She attended all the parties that week and bid day finally came. Bid day is when the sorority members vote and choose the girls they would like to have in their sorority. Then you get to decide which one you want to join based on which of the sororities chose you. It was common knowledge in this small college every girl was rushed by all three sororities so it really came down to the girls choosing which one they liked most.

She had made her choice. There was one she desperately wanted to be a part of. The big day came for her to go to the office, listen to the director tell her she had been selected by all three and then profoundly declare her choice.

The director smiled with that "let's see" smile while she opened the first box of bids and began thumbing through them. As she neared the back of the box, the look grew to one of confusion. She hadn't seen my friend's name in there. She quickly grabbed the second box of bids. As she combed through this one she commented on how she must have missed it, so she combed back through them with a very confused and almost embarrassed look on her face. Her smile was fading and so was this beautiful young woman's. The director quickly grabbed the third box, the sorority that my friend had desperately wanted to join all along, and then almost shouted out with relief when she found her name in the file.

With a shallow thank you, my friend took the card and turned to walk out with her head looking down toward the ground. This was the sorority she had so desperately wanted to join but suddenly she was feeling dejected and rejected by not being selected by the other two. She began asking herself, why didn't they want me? The other girls got bids from all three. Why hadn't I?

As the years went on, the bright, vibrant woman became quiet and shy. At work she wouldn't socialize with the other women. At home she stayed to herself and never participated in outside activities. It came time for her to interview for a higher position in her company. When she discovered it was a female who would be interviewing her, she was riddled with anxiety. After all, all those other girls had rejected her.

One day after going through a personal growth program, she was able to identify how much the incident in college had impacted her life and kept her stuck in her cocoon of a comfort zone. She never wanted to feel that type of pain and rejection ever again. She had formed the belief about herself that she wasn't worthy and not good enough for those other girls in the other two sororities.

After going through this discovery, she was back in her hometown visiting and she ran into one of the leaders from one of the sororities who "didn't want her." This time she had grown personally and so she asked the woman, "Why did y'all not choose me?"

For 30 years she had lived in the belief she created that they had not wanted her. For 30 years she had avoided becoming friends with other women. For 30 years she had been wrong. The woman looked at her and answered with this: "Oh my, we really wanted you and so did the other sorority, but your sorority wanted you SO BAD they came to both of us and begged us please not to bid on you. We honored that because we knew you wanted them too and we didn't want you to turn us down." For 30 years those "bees" of belief had buzzed around in my friend's head, and she had listened to them. Now, 30 years later, she was starting to live again and making friends with other women. She won't be held back by the buzzing bees ever again.

What have you missed out on in your life because of the beliefs you have created about yourself based on someone else's opinion? Or beliefs you created from stories you made up in your mind based on something you believed to be true? I know how easily it can happen. I made a lot of mistakes in my life based on beliefs I had about myself that were based on my interpretation of what someone else said, did or didn't say.

At some point you get to decide how long you want to hold onto those beliefs that keep you stuck in the comfort zone you are in. Now you might claim that where you are is not a comfortable place, but I'm just saying – you wouldn't still be there if it wasn't!

Here's the thing, if you own those beliefs, you get to be right about not being smart enough, not being good enough, just NOT BEING. There's a pay-off in that and even if you say you don't like being that way or feeling that way, the truth is, it's comfortable and you are staying 10 feet from the edge of something.

So how do you change it?

Step 1:

LET GO OF THE EMOTIONAL ATTACHMENT

Write down all those things you believe to be true. Write down all those "bees" buzzing in your ears. It may be hard and it may get emotional, so pick a PRIVATE time and place to just write down your feelings about the pain – let yourself feel the emotion.

What are the things that happened to you to make you form those beliefs? Maybe you were molested by a family member or a friend as a child and you blamed yourself. Maybe a parent was physically or verbally abusive and you believed you were not worthy of love or acceptance. Maybe you were abandoned at birth by your parents, and although you had great adoptive parents, you had this underlying belief you were not good enough to be loved – at least not by the one person who was supposed to love you the most. Or maybe you spent your entire life trying to please your adoptive parents so they wouldn't throw you away too.

Maybe you were raped as a young teen and you believed it was your fault for wearing a skirt that was too short or that you were somewhere you shouldn't have been and your loved ones said that to you. Maybe it was someone you trusted or looked up to that committed the crime. Maybe, like my friend, you weren't "chosen" for something you really wanted. Ask yourself and write down the answers to those things you are clinging to. Only by accepting them as roadblocks can you release them.

Step 2:

MAKE A LIST

In list format, write down the beliefs you have been holding onto about yourself. Put a face on the "bee" – or the bee-lief – either a real person or a fictional character. There may be more than one "bee" buzzing in your ear. Draw the face on it or paste a picture on the "bee's" face. Make copies of the "bee" pictured at the end of this chapter and name each one by writing the belief under the picture of the 'bee'.

Step 3:

NAME IT!

Put a face and/or a name beside each "bee"… the bee-lief.

Example:

I'm not smart enough.   PERCEPTION

I'm not pretty enough.   JOE

I'm lazy. ATTITUDE

Step 4:

LET GO

Pick a date and time to let the "bees" go.

Step 5:

SQUASH THE "BEES"!

At the chosen time on the chosen date, SQUASH THE "BEES"! Just kidding, but do something symbolic to take back your power.

Stomp on the pictures, shred them, bottle them up with a tight cap and throw them away, burn them and scatter the ashes … whatever works for you. Maybe you buy a stuffed bee, pull out the stuffing and re-stuff it with the shreds and sew it back up. I know it sounds crazy, but sometimes we just need to do something symbolic to take back our power. It may be that you just need to sit down face-to-face and ask the questions you need to ask.

Step 6:

FORGIVE & LET GO

- Forgive them
- Forgive yourself for allowing them to steal your power.
- Be grateful to yourself for the letting go.

YOU ARE WORTH IT!!

And the next time you begin to hear a faint buzzing in your ear, shoo it away immediately and don't go there! You are worth it. You are worthy of all that you desire your life to be. Move over to the edge and step out of your comfort zone. Step over that edge and start living the life you deserve.

It's a

GREAT DAY

and

YOU ARE

a

beautiful person!

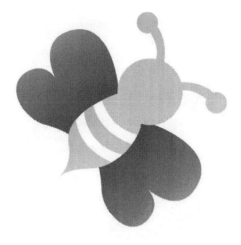

NAME YOUR *"Bee"* _____

What is the BEE-lief you had about yourself that is keeping you stuck in your comfort zone or holding you back in life?

_____

_____

_____

_____

_____

_____

_____

Date & Time to release it?

_____

"Success
is when you work hard to better yourself.
Significance
is when you work hard to better others."

- JOHN C. MAXWELL

Chapter 11

Success
vs.
Significance

John C. Maxwell is known as the "leadership guru" of the world. Do a search on Amazon, Google or You Tube. He is one of the most internationally respected and highly regarded authors and experts on leadership and personal and professional development, and I am on his team. He is one of my mentors.

Being a part of The John Maxwell Team has been a great gift in my life. It came at a time where I was looking for that "next step" to grow forward and live into my true purpose and vision. I have been an admirer of John C. Maxwell for many years and have always loved his books on leadership and personal growth. Never in my wildest dreams before a few years ago did I believe I would end up becoming a coach on his speaking, training and coaching team.

On January 23, 2012, when I sat in the auditorium in Pensacola, Florida to hear John speak, I had no idea it would become another defining moment in my life. I was searching for something. All my working adult life I have said I wanted to be a keynote inspirational speaker. I love the stage and I love delivering a message that challenges others to think, to reflect and to get out of their comfort zone when they are stuck. Whether it is sales, leadership, or just sharing my story, I love inspiring others to grow beyond where they ever thought possible.

Have you ever had one of those moments in life where you just knew you were supposed to do something? That feeling in your gut that is so strong you have to act on it? This was one of those times. As they spoke of the team they had formed to help carry on John's vision, I knew I had been given those tickets for a reason.

I believe in fate, and just a few days before the event, a friend who was on my team with the national health and wellness company I have worked with over the last 10 years mentioned she was going and had two extra tickets. I jumped at the chance. I was there that day as an answer to prayers.

We get our answer every time, but often we don't respond to it. We question it or decide that was not really the answer we were looking for. I am blessed with an intuitive nature I've learned to listen to. Sometimes it is almost like it hits me over the head, it comes so strong. At the end of John's talk, they offered for people to stay after if they wanted to learn more about becoming a member of the team. My husband, Bill, was with me, and it clearly was NOT his vision for himself – it wasn't even his vision for me!

He was ready to leave, but I knew I had to stay, so he left and went out to wait in the car. I didn't let that concern me because I knew I was supposed to hear this. I knew before they even told me anything about it that I would be a part of it. I just didn't know how.

The company I had worked with for eight years had just gone bankrupt, and I had not had a paycheck for a few months. I had gone from making a LOT of money to making NO money, and we had gone through what savings we had. I needed to find my next step in life. I remember hearing a quote at the age of 15 that stuck with me through life. "Where there's a will, there's a way." I had the will, and I would find the way.

I am not a "religious" person, but I am a very spiritual person. I am a firm believer that when God has a plan for us, he also creates the circumstances for that plan to come to fruition. If we are smart, we will notice those moments and seize them. So I stepped out in faith and committed to what I knew was His plan for me, and I am so glad I did.

My mentors on the team have challenged me to grow in a powerful way. They helped me find my passion again. I have loved every one of my coaching clients, my corporate clients and my speaking engagements, and with each, I have grown that much more. I get the opportunity to see a lot of people who, like I once was, are 10 feet from the edge and stuck in their comfort zone. I have also had the opportunity to support them in moving past that.

There has been one other time in the last couple of years I got that same gut feeling I had the day I watched John Maxwell speak in Pensacola, Florida. It was at the John Maxwell Team certification training in February 2013. It was the day I heard him speak about an opportunity for helping to create positive change in the country of Guatemala. He spoke of taking a team there for a Transformational Leadership mission trip. I wrote on my paper as he spoke about his journey and meetings with every leader in Guatemala: "I am going to Guatemala." There was no doubt in my mind. He had not said where he would get the team from or who he would take, but I knew!

This story has been such an impactful and important part of my recent journey, I would be remiss not to share at least a small vision of it in this book. Actually, it is a book all in itself, but I will summarize the most impactful moments down to one (longer) chapter here.

It was April before they announced John was accepting applications from the John Maxwell Team mentorship group. Once again, I didn't know how, but I knew I was called to be there. And yes, when He has a plan, it just happens.

I filled out my application and was blessed to be accepted to be a part of the team of 150 coaches from around the world that would travel with John Maxwell to Guatemala. It was one of the most game-changing experiences of my life. It was the time that I truly understood the difference between success and significance. As John says in his book, *Becoming a Person of Influence:*

"*Success*
is when you work hard to better yourself.

Significance
is when you work hard to better others."

We experienced significance on that journey. It changed the lives of every single person who was fortunate enough to go. It also changed the lives of more than 20,000 Guatemalan leaders and will continue to change lives as those leaders ripple what they learned out to hundreds of thousands of others in their impoverished country. Many trainers and speakers can say they were a part of transforming a company; however, I still pinch myself when I think about the fact I was an integral part of transforming a COUNTRY.

On my flight from Atlanta to Guatemala, I was given a hint of just how significant the journey would be. I had the privilege of sitting next to a young Guatemalan businessman. I was asking him about his family, his business and his country. Now let me sidestep here for just moment to tell you that I speak NO Spanish ... NONE! I had ordered a program that would teach you to speak Spanish in 10 days about two months before I left. It arrived at my home the day before I left! I never even had time to open it.

Fortunately, my new friend José spoke very good English. He asked me why I was coming to Guatemala and I asked if he knew who John Maxwell was. His eyes lit up and he said, "YES! I love Mr. Maxwell. I have read his books!" I explained to him that I was part of his coaching team and that we were coming there to train 20,000 Guatemalan business, faith, government, educational, military and family leaders on a Transformational Leadership program called *La Transformacion Esta En Mi*. In English that translates to something like "transformation begins in me."

As I spoke of our mission to train 20,000 on how to facilitate the same program throughout the country, my new friend had tears in his eyes. He looked at me and said with a heartfelt voice, "Thank you, Peggy, thank you. My country needs you." My heart melted. I knew that the next week was going down in the book of significance.

We arrived in Guatemala City about noon on Monday, and we would meet with John Maxwell at two that afternoon to learn about our mission. The funny thing? We didn't even know what was going to take place really. We went on faith and knowledge that we were supposed to be there and that God had a plan for that week. And it was a darn good thing because nobody else did!

Joking aside, the coordinators really were still putting it all together when we arrived as it had taken on a life of its own and grown significantly larger than they had originally expected. We would be working in conjunction with EQUIP (a Maxwell Company), a wonderful Guatemalan non-profit organization, Guatemala Prospera, and some longtime friends of John's with a company called La Red Business Network, which has a values-based curriculum.

Our mission was to teach some 20,000 Guatemalan leaders how to facilitate a 30-week, values-based, round-table program. Fifteen of the values we would provide came from a needs survey of more than 12,000 Guatemalans, and 15 came from John's book on The 15 Invaluable Laws of Growth.

I shared my airplane story with John when we arrived at the meeting place. He had tears in his eyes as he thanked me for sharing it. It added such value for him to hear how important locals thought this would be to their country and that the fruits of all his hard work would be worthwhile.

We learned that our schedule would consist of teaching us how to facilitate the program on Monday and Tuesday, then Wednesday practicing with our interpreters and Thursday, Friday and Saturday actually training the leaders. It would culminate with a stadium event on Saturday afternoon and then a big private celebration hosted by John on Saturday night in Antigua.

Oh, and did I mention we would be the guests of the President of Guatemala at his palace on Wednesday night? He wanted to thank each of us for being there for his country. It was a powerful night to witness as he spoke of the opportunities this would bring his country and how much he would support its continuation.

Working with the interpreters on Wednesday was really stretching my comfort zone. Learning to speak in sound bites followed by someone repeating your words in another language was, well, challenging. But it was also a GREAT experience. I was so impressed with all the interpreters who were volunteering their time.

Many of them were from the local college, and interpreting was a course major for them. Some of them had done this many times before and so they were very helpful in teaching us how to work with an interpreter. Some of them were just as new to interpreting as we were, so we learned together. I loved the two young men I was practicing with and had hoped to get to work with them that week, but that didn't turn out to be the case.

The businesses and groups we would be training were broken up into groups of approximately 40 each. The coordinating team had worked all night figuring out who would go where on Thursday morning – matching coaches with groups and interpreters with coaches. Some coaches would train with a partner and one interpreter and some would train solo with an interpreter. As hard as they worked, there was still a LOT of confusion because word had spread quickly and so many people in Guatemala wanted to participate, and they were just showing up to get on the list. It was a great problem to have but we clearly needed to find a new system!

Thursday

Thursday and Friday were broken into two training sessions – one in the morning and one in the afternoon. I was assigned to train solo that first morning. I was SO excited, so nervous, and just trusting that it would happen just the way it was supposed to. God likes to play tricks sometimes when we need to move past our fears and grow. He presented me with my own "growth opportunity" that very first training day.

At first I got out to my bus to find that I did not have an interpreter. My interpreter was assigned and already partnered up with someone else. Yes, the girl who received her *How to Speak Spanish* course the day before she left on this foreign journey had no interpreter. They grabbed a very polished looking man and said, "You go with her!" I should have known I was in for trouble when he walked on in his polished casual look but had a hang-up bag with a suit in it so he could dress to match the person he would be supporting. (Actually, I think he wanted to be sure he could outshine the person with whom he would be working!)

He introduced himself and quickly let me know he was a professional interpreter. That wasn't all he let me know! He first let me know our translation of *La Transformacion Esta En Mi* was incorrect, which sent up the first red flag. He was a "know-it-all." Literally, he was brilliant. However, he wanted to establish up front how he was going to do things. We would take a break when HE was ready, and his way was not in line with how we were coached to facilitate or how I practiced with an interpreter.

It was time for my leadership skills to be put to the test! The first group I would facilitate was a leadership team from Ban Rural, one of the largest banks in Guatemala. When we arrived, my interpreter wanted to go change into the suit he brought along since I was more professionally dressed in a suit. I made it clear to Mr. Know-it-all we would take a break when the bank manager was ready. However, I decided to stretch and agree to try his way on the interpreting thing (even though I knew with my A.D.D. someone talking at the same time I was would be a REAL challenge!)

He wanted me to just talk and he would talk right behind me in Spanish – no sound bites. On top of my talking. I am just here to tell you – that did NOT work for me! And it did not work for the audience. Fortunately, one of the class members raised their hand to say they were having a difficult time following him while I was speaking. YES! Mr. Know-it-all didn't know it all! So we shifted and went back to my way. I wanted to say, they are not paying me enough to put up with this guy, but then I remembered they weren't paying me at all! I don't think I mentioned that part. The 150 coaches all paid their own expenses to come help with this transformational mission trip. It was worth every penny.

After we got through that bumpy start it was smooth sailing. The group loved the program and they participated in all the exercises. They were so eager and willing to learn and they felt so blessed we were there. One of the other facilitators was training a second group in another room, so we joined together in the end to give them their certificates. When we were finished, they each came up one-by-one to hug us and say thank you. After four hours of training, that day was done but my lessons weren't.

After the bus (did I say armed guard bus?) returned to the hotel, I invited my interpreter to join me and share my lunch. We were together by design that day. We each needed to learn lessons from each other and we spent the next three hours in amazing conversation about life and challenges and growth. As it turned out, the Mr. Know-it-all facade was just a cover for a very insecure man. I coached him through gray areas he saw as black and white and we shared very personal stories that connected us on a deep level. God knew what he was doing.

My first day as a facilitator in Guatemala was powerful.

Friday

The amazing leadership team did come up with a new plan for getting us out the next morning. Have you ever heard that saying "K.I.S.S. – Keep it simple, stupid"? They went back to simplicity and so we all arrived at 6:30 a.m., not knowing or caring if we would be on the morning or the afternoon team or both. We just knew "we were going somewhere, at some time, with somebody – just go with the flow." It became our theme for the week.

Flexibility has always been a strong suit of mine, so I was cool with that. It was fun, however, to watch those who were very scheduled and detailed walk into the unknown and to see how much growth came from just that experience. It was definitely a lesson in flexibility for that group and a lesson on how my scheduled clients may feel when I put them in similar situations!

WOO HOO! I was in the morning group! I had not missed all those extra hours of sleep I could have had to find out I wasn't needed until the afternoon. It was a simple process. When your table is called, go through this line to get your training materials and get in this line to be matched up with an interpreter on your way out the door to get in whatever car pulled up next. They had offered us the opportunity to pair up with the same interpreter we had the day before but I was open to finding a new one!

On Wednesday afternoon after we had worked with the interpreters, I saw a beautiful Guatemalan woman standing over by herself. I went up and introduced myself to Marisella. She had such a quiet, glowing spirit about her.

I learned that she was a well-educated technical engineer with a tremendous background in internet technology. She had been laid off from her job many months before and had been unable to find another one. She had come to help on blind faith without even having the money for gas to get home. She had heard of the opportunity as an interpreter for this transformation program through her church and she just knew, like me, she was called to be there.

I offered to have her parking garage ticket stamped since I was a hotel guest, and since I had not spent the quetzals (Guatemalan money) I had exchanged at the airport, I gave her some of that. Truthfully, I didn't even know how much I gave her but she seemed really grateful and happy. I just knew by the schedule, I was not going to have time to spend it before I left!

We went over to the hotel and visited for a while. I remember her asking me "Why did you choose me? Why did you come up and talk with me?" The hardship of losing her job and going for months interviewing and getting no job had really taken a toll on her self-esteem. She had formed beliefs about herself based on False Evidence Appearing Real.

I told her what I saw was a beautiful woman with a warm, inviting smile, and I wanted to know her story. I wish I had time in this book to share with you the many lessons she taught me over the next few days. We still stay in contact today. She is truly a child of God with the most beautiful spirit I have ever seen. She is so talented in so many areas and she is the face of some of the biggest challenges Guatemalans face. She had had success, but this week she would experience significance.

So on Thursday morning, we partnered up to go out on our adventure. Our assignment was to train the leaders and attorneys in the government judicial system. I was amazed to find that all the attorneys were in there twenties. We had a great training. We laughed a lot, we shed some tears together as people opened up during the values lessons and we learned a lot from each other. Again, they were SO grateful for us being there and bringing this to them. If only they truly understood the gift it was to me to be able to share this with them.

Marisella and I arrived back at the hotel just after noon exhausted from the heat and four hours on our feet pouring everything we had into these hungry, eager-to-learn leaders. We plopped down with our stuff, shared a lunch and stories of the morning while we cooled down. I was done for the day, and it was a good thing because I was spent!

And then it happened. God said, "Nope! You are not done with your lessons for the day – there is a much bigger experience you need to have." About two, John's personal interpreter came to me in the lobby with a look of desperation on his face. He said, "Peggy, we have a group that has been waiting on a facilitator for an hour and we have no one to send them. Do you know anyone who could go?"

Now he was saying this as he was getting down on his knees by my chair and speaking in that almost begging voice. I looked at him and I said, "Yes. I will go. I have all my materials here with me (I had not even gone up to my room to put things away yet). Where am I going?" He told me he had one of the interpreters from Guatemala Prospera who would be going with me. So I said goodbye to Marisella and grabbed my bag to go.

I haven't told you yet about the warnings we had in the beginning. Don't go ANYWHERE by yourself – always in groups of five or more, don't take your cell phone out in public, don't wear jewelry, blend in, only keep a few dollars visible or on you at all. Gangs of bad guys would come up to your car or bus with guns while you were stopped at a red light to steal your phones and money. It is an everyday occurrence throughout the country.

Most of the buses we were transported on had armed guards on them and there were armed military on every corner in Guatemala City. Every facility we pulled up to had locked gates with armed guards. It was an eye-opening experience, and that was in the capital city.

So we go out to meet our ride to the awaiting group. I had to walk around a small, old, beat-up car sitting in front of the doors to the hotel. I was looking around for the bus or van that would transport us. Suddenly I heard someone call my name and I turned to see my interpreter walking toward that old car

I had just walked around. She said "This is our ride! I will let you get in the front seat."

Now you have to understand, I was living in my fear zone based on everything we had been told. As I sat down in this car with no windows, and a hole where the radio had obviously been stolen from, I thought to myself, yep this is it. I am going to die today.

Thank goodness I was not in my bright coral suit jacket from the day before in the 100-degree heat sticking out like a sore thumb saying, "Come rob us! She doesn't belong here!" My survival mode stepped in, so I took my cell phone and rammed it up under my bottom and stuck my money down my bra and away we went!

Traffic was horrendous, and we were stopped for long periods of time. It took us 30 minutes to get to our destination only a few miles away. During that time, and through my interpreter, I found out that I would be training the heads of all sports in the country from the Sports Federation.

This powerful group of mostly men had now been waiting for an hour and a half when I arrived. You can imagine their level of tolerance at this point. These were important leaders who were told to be in this room. They really didn't even understand fully what it was they were there for. I almost felt I was walking into a somewhat hostile environment.

My training from John Maxwell's book *Everyone Communicates*

Few Connect came in handy that day. I quickly found a way to connect with several of them by sharing some brief funny experiences with their sport. They loved my canoe story with my girlfriends and the story of my first golf outing with my now husband when we were dating.

He and one of the guys I worked with at the time put their ball in the water on the first hole, and I put my "practice ball from the men's tee" on the green. My husband says his worst nightmare came true in that moment. That ended our golf outings but they both felt vindicated when the large pelican pooped on my head midways through the game!

So after we laughed a little and all loosened up, I began to share the purpose of our journey to Guatemala and what *La Transformacion Esta En Mi* was all about. When we began the process of learning how to facilitate the program I asked for three volunteers. It was like pulling teeth, but then one-by-one three of the men came to the front to volunteer.

The roundtable process begins with taking turns reading the lesson so those three got the easy part. The others gained confidence and thought well this is easy, so getting my next set of volunteers was a little quicker. That group, however, got to answer some thought-provoking questions about what they had just learned. To my surprise, they really began opening up and sharing.

With the next topic, I had no problem getting the first three volunteers. This entire process was about change and how living these values and laws of growth could help facilitate that change. As the facilitator, I had shared some brief personal stories of times in my life I experienced fear of change. This allowed them to open up and share as well.

We were running along smoothly, and then it was break time. They had a spread of food in the back, but since we had started late and I wanted to honor their time, I asked what length of break they wanted. One gentleman quickly said "Let's take five minutes and get our food and continue while we eat so we can get out of here on time." I got that he was not 100% engaged – the tough nut to crack so to speak.

During the break one of the very well-dressed, distinguished leaders came to me and in a heartfelt voice of broken English said, "Thank you, Peggy, thank you for sharing your heart and your story of being on your own with three daughters. I too have just gone through a divorce and found myself on my own with three girls, and now I have hope in listening to your story." He gave me a hug and I thanked him, and then we went back to our training program. We never know the impact a brief story can have on a person.

As we neared the end of our training time, I knew I had one last chance to impact the "tougher nuts" in the room. As exhausted and hot as I was, I dug deep to share the passion I felt for this project.

I spoke of success and I spoke of significance. I spoke of the far reaching power this program would have in the country. I reminded them of the tremendous gift each would experience and the impact it could have on the success of their sports teams, their families and their friends.

I looked at each as I told them, "You will be able to say – I was in the room the week the transformation of my country began. I was a significant part of this historical moment in the great transformation of my country."

As I finished my passionate, heartfelt speech I opened the floor for questions. The "tough nut" to crack ... the one who wanted the short break ... began to speak. He started out thanking me for the valuable material and insight. I was beginning to feel warm and fuzzy. Then it happened. Suddenly he raised his workbook and proclaimed, in his version of English, "However, if this has ANYTHING to do with politica (politics) I'll have NO part of it!" With that, he slammed his book down on the table and stared at me with that "What do you have to say now?" look.

WELL – OK! How you gonna handle this one? I just knew the can of worms was now open and this could be my nightmare. Would they all jump on his bandwagon? Panic was setting in and I was trying to figure out how I would turn THIS one around.

That ride in that open, beat up little car across town didn't seem near as frightening now! I was about to be attacked by 30-plus heads of competitive sports teams. And I couldn't even speak the language!

Suddenly something amazing happened. My friend who had connected with my story stood up. He said "This is a round table and it is safe for me to share. Three days ago myself, a Jewish friend and a Muslim friend and my friend visiting from England all gathered together. I have been through much hardship, and like Peggy, I have been through a divorce with three children and my business has been failing. Together we fell to our knees and prayed that God would bring something that could change our country and my situation." At that moment he turned to me, raised his hand toward me and profoundly proclaimed "TODAY YOU ARE HERE!"

He continued to look to Mr. Tough Nut and say "I don't care if politica is involved. This is about me. This is about the future of my family and my country! *La Transformacion Esta En Mi!* With that, he sat down.

About this time tears were welling up inside of me. My interpreter was standing right behind me with her chin on my shoulder translating in my ear as if she were quietly commenting on a golf or tennis match. Then it happened again.

The next man rose to his feet and began to share a story about how his seven-year-old daughter had been diagnosed with bone cancer with no hope to live. He shared how his church had come together to pay for them to go to America to St. Jude's Children's hospital in Tennessee.

As tears streamed down his face, and mine by this time, he shared how they had been given a second chance at life when it was determined that in fact she only had a small removable tumor and what was in her bones was only an infection that was treatable. He looked at Mr. Tough Nut and with a raised voice proclaimed "THIS IS NOT ABOUT POLITICA. THIS IS ABOUT MY DAUGHTER'S FUTURE. THIS IS ABOUT MY COUNTRY'S FUTURE!"

By now, my interpreter was crying so hard she could barely translate. My shoulder was soaked with her tears and the front of my shirt with mine. Then another stood and spoke of how his best friend had just died that day, and he should have been with him and his family at the funeral home. But he was here with us because "I can't do anything to bring my friend back, but I can honor him and all others by being a part of the transformation of my country. I can honor him by bringing these values and laws to his family and his children and I can honor myself by living these."

After a couple others spoke, the man sitting next to Mr. Tough Nut turned to him and began to speak. (I am sure by now he wanted to crawl under the table and suck every one of the words he said back inside.) His counterpart turned to him and pointed at him as he spoke in a stern yet steady voice. He said "My friend, YOU ARE WRONG! This is NOT about politica! I WAS IN THE ROOM when John Maxwell first came to our country. I was in the room when leaders who wanted to see change in our country came together to speak with him of how this could happen. This was all before he ever met with the president. You are wrong my friend. This is about ME...this is about YOU and THIS is about saving OUR COUNTRY!

La Transformacion Esta En Mi and in YOU!"

Everyone had tears in their eyes. In that moment, everyone experienced significance. Their lives would change forever. My life changed forever that night.

I didn't even care that we were driving back to our hotel in an old, beat-up car with the windows out. God had touched my life in a powerful way that afternoon. I will be forever grateful He chose me to be with that group. When I arrived back at the hotel it was already after seven. I had finished on time, but they told stories for over an hour and NO ONE left.

My team was already upstairs eating dinner, and somehow I found the strength to walk up to join them. As I sat down at one of the only seats left, I remember just staring around the room. The realization of the significance of what we were doing suddenly overwhelmed me. Tears began to fall down my cheeks. We stood to sing and have the blessing and I wept.

The girl across the table noticed I was crying and asked if I was OK. I looked at her and shook my head and said "I don't know. What I just experienced was so powerful, so life changing, I don't know. I am so full of love, appreciation and gratitude. I now know what John meant when he said this week you will know the difference in success and significance."

My tablemates all asked me to please share what had happened. I was almost too numb to tell the story of the transformation I had just witnessed. But I did. It was why we were there. I now understood what my friend on the airplane meant when he said "my country needs you". I now understood the meaning of *La Transformacion Esta En Mi!*

" Create adventures in your life that stretch your comfort zone. Live into your purpose, your passion and step-by-step,

walk up to the edge

and step over into your possibilities. "

Chapter 12

And *Life* Grows On

Over the years there would be many challenges to life, but that's just life, isn't it? We all go through challenges and as the saying goes, "What doesn't kill you makes you stronger." I like to say I GROW through challenges instead of just going through them. Shoot, I have grown so tall I have a hard time getting through the door!

So now you know my story. The story of the choices I made during those tough times. Here is what I can tell you: I wouldn't be the person I am today had I not gone through that and made the choices I did.

My life will never be "normal" according to others' standards, but it is my "normal." I am reminded daily as I use my catheter to drain the pouch, as I carefully choose the foods I can eat, that I am thankful. Thankful for the gift of life and for what is "normal" for me. I am thankful that God gave me the right to choose how I live each and every day of my life. It will never be simple.

As of this writing, I have had more than 15 surgeries, and right now I am waiting to choose the right time for the next one to repair my sixth hernia. Each time it is a little harder, but I have the most wonderful life partner now, my husband, Bill Brockman. He has been through at least six or seven of those surgeries with me.

Six months after we were married, I had a total revision of the internal pouch to convert it from a Kock Pouch to an improved Barnett Continent Intestinal Reservoir (BCIR) at Palms of

Pasadena Hospital in St. Petersburg, Florida. Dr. James Pollack did that surgery and the procedure is typically a 21 day hospital stay. I made it through that one with flying colors and no complications. Once again, my family was there for me.

Bill is my strength each time even though it is never easy for him. He worries so much about me, but I will be OK. I choose to be a survivor and to keep it in perspective and stay positive about the gifts I have been given and the gifts I am able to give as a result. YOU get to choose how you handle the challenges in your life.

CHOOSE
to
Live & *Grow*
FULLY
through them.

Each day when you put your feet on the floor, choose the attitude you want for that day. If you wake up and stub your toe and decide it is going to be a bad day, it will be. If you change your thought process and realize it is only one little tiny moment of your day and it will pass, then it will.

Let it Go!

Let me ask you some self-assessment questions that may take you out of your comfort zone to answer:

• What are the things you need to let go of in life that keep you 10 feet from the edge of having what you truly want?

_____

_____

_____

_____

_____

_____

• What are the things that keep you stuck in your comfort zone?

_____

_____

_____

_____

_____

_____

• Do you really want to move forward or have you gotten so comfortable you just want to curl up and stay there?

_____

_____

_____

_____

_____

• What kind of attitude do you think you have?

_____

_____

_____

_____

_____

• What kind of attitude would others say you have?

_____

_____

_____

_____

_____

• When something bad happens, what is your first reaction?

_____

_____

_____

_____

_____

_____

• Do you love to get caught up in the drama of it all?

_____

_____

_____

_____

• What do you believe to be the truths about you?

_____

_____

_____

_____

• What are the Bee-liefs you have been holding onto and for how long?

_____

_____

_____

_____

_____

_____

_____

_____

_____

_____

_____

• When do you want to let go of them?

_____

_____

_____

_____

• What are you avoiding?

_____

_____

_____

_____

_____

_____

_____

_____

_____

• What holds you back?

_____

_____

_____

_____

_____

_____

_____

_____

• Who do you want to be?

_____

_____

_____

_____

_____

_____

_____

_____

_____

_____

• What is your purpose?

_____

_____

_____

_____

_____

_____

_____

_____

_____

• Do you have a vision for your life?

_____

_____

_____

_____

• What is your vision?

_____

_____

_____

_____

_____

_____

_____

_____

_____

• Do you regularly set goals for yourself?

_____

_____

_____

• What are your top three life goals?

_____

_____

_____

_____

_____

_____

_____

_____

_____

_____

_____

• What do you believe in?

_____

_____

_____

_____

_____

_____

• Are willing to commit to change?

_____

_____

_____

• How will you benefit by changing?

_____

_____

_____

_____

_____

_____

_____

_____

_____

_____

_____

_____

_____

_____

My hope is that in some way, my stories have made a difference in your life and challenged you in some small way or some big way to step outside your comfort zone. I continue to challenge myself every day. Any time I feel like I am getting a little stuck in life, or I feel fearful, I do something that jolts me out of that stuck place. My commitment is to keep doing that.

Over the years, after my rappelling adventure, I have done many things to take me way outside my comfort zone. I don't know that I will ever completely eliminate my fear of heights or the fact that I get claustrophobic. I use the excuse that it runs in my family. However, I challenge myself continually to break free from those fears and false truths.

Prior to one of my surgeries that I was feeling uneasy about, I made my husband take me hang-gliding the day before I went into the hospital. Bless his heart (as we would say in the South), he had just had knee replacement surgery eight weeks before, but he knew it was something I needed to do. I knew if I could do that I could make it through the surgery and the recovery time I would face. It was another one of those exhilarating feelings of "YES, I can do this!"

In 2004, I was blessed with the opportunity to become an Honorary Commander of the 33rd Fighter Wing at Eglin Air Force Base. They select a handful of community leaders each year to serve a full year learning about the Air Force and bridging the gap between our military community and the civilian community.

It was one of the most meaningful years of my life. I truly learned what they meant by "military family". At the end of my year, I was blessed with the opportunity to take a flight in an F-15 Fighter Jet. It was an honor very few civilians ever receive.

I remember the day so vividly. I put on my flight suit and Colonel Ron "Ernie" Banks, my squadron commander, escorted me to the flight line and assisted me in climbing up into the back seat of the cockpit. I could hear my teeth chattering. I was filled with excitement, gratitude and yes, a LOT of anxiousness, all right – FEAR if I want to be honest – about this flight.

As we revved up the engines, there was an issue that needed to be repaired so we climbed back out of the jet and we waited another 45 minutes or so. That was actually good for me because when I got back in, I already knew what that seat felt like and I knew what to do, or at least I thought I did.

As we revved up the engines for the second time and began taxiing down the runway, I had that same feeling of when I was standing on that ledge at Cheaha State Park some 12 years earlier. Suddenly we were in full throttle take-off, and then we turned and went straight up in to the air with after burners blasting.

And that is when it happened. The G-suit began inflating and everything I had been taught went straight out of my mind. I saw the grey closing in and all I could remember was my girlfriend who had taken a flight told me that she just began shouting out something and the blood came back to her head. About that time I screamed out something like, "Oh my gosh! ... Holy geez!" (I don't think my words were quite that nice!)

I think I scared poor Ernie to death! He quickly throttled back so we weren't pulling as many G's and all was good, until he started doing the aileron rolls and we were upside down and all around.

If you know anything about F-15's, they have a glass canopy top. I remember looking out from hundreds of feet in the air and really appreciating the beauty of the world below, until he made that one turn that got my stomach. Fortunately I had my Ziploc bags handy – it was a two-bagger flight for me!

An F-15 is not the best place for someone who is claustrophobic (you have on all the head gear and mask as well as a G-suit that inflates when you pull G's) or has a fear of heights (you are hundreds of feet in the air with a glass canopy top,) but it was the best place for me. It was the best place for me to stretch my comfort zone to a whole new level.

Not many civilians can say they've flown in an F-15. I got to actually hold that stick and fly that bad boy, and it was a feeling of control like no other. I can honestly say, it was a once in a life time opportunity, and one I only want to do once!

Nothing will compare to that, but just last year, I was feeling a little overwhelmed and stuck, so I went zip-lining in Honduras. My husband must really love me. He goes along with me on these crazy adventures.

I also had the honor of serving as an Honorary Commander for the 1st Special OPS Group at Hurlburt Field, and we got to sit on the open aft ramp and cargo door (or the tail gate as I called it — and yes, they laughed at me) of an MC-130H Combat Talon II. Tethered in, we dangled our feet over the edge and marveled at the beautiful view in the open air as we flew a few hundred feet above the beautiful Gulf Coast.

I hope you will create adventures in your life that stretch your comfort zone. Live into your purpose, your passion, and step-by-step, walk up to the edge and step over into your possibilities. And if you ever get really stuck, contact me! I know a great coach who's been there!

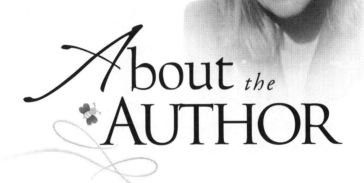

About the AUTHOR

Peggy Brockman

As an inspirational speaker, author, and a respected member of John C. Maxwell's international speaking, training and coaching team, Peggy Brockman has moved thousands of people around the world to improve their lives, step OUT of old comfort zones and reach beyond their expectations. She delivers RELEVANT, game-changing solutions based on real-life EXPERIENCE, fundamental RESEARCH, and the kind of PERSPECTIVE and INSIGHT that help propel today's audiences to make the CHANGE and CHOICES necessary to WIN with character, humor and a sense of balance.

Peggy has been an entrepreneur since the age of 25. She has an extensive background in sales and sales management both in the media world and the network marketing/direct sales industry. She made it to the top of a network marketing company and led a team of over 2,000 consultants. Peggy traveled the country training thousands of people on how to be successful sales entrepreneurs. She has inspired audiences of up to 5,000 people from the stage and has entertained even larger audiences as a television show host and a radio show host. Peggy owned a personal and professional development school and modeling and acting school and agency for many years before moving to Florida. Once in Florida, she went in to media sales and corporate management, managing a local television station. She has also been on the founding boards for two non-profit organizations – an agency against domestic violence and an arts foundation.

Peggy also passionately serves her local community in many leadership capacities including American Business Women's

Association, American Society for Training and Development, Referral Leaders International and the Panhandle Animal Welfare Society. She is a former Chair of the Board of the Greater Fort Walton Beach, Florida Chamber of Commerce and the annual Peggy Brockman Leadership Award was established in her honor by Leadership Okaloosa (County) in 2005. She has also served as a civilian Honorary Commander for the 33rd Fighter Wing at Eglin Air Force Base and the 1st Special OPS Group at Hurlburt Field. Peggy is married to the love of her life, Bill, and they live in Ft. Walton Beach, Florida. They have five beautiful daughters and seven amazing grandchildren around the country.

Whether you are looking for a DYNAMIC SPEAKER to MOTIVATE your group or you want to take advantage of Peggy's vast knowledge in the personal and professional DEVELOPMENT realm or her SALES and LEADERSHIP expertise – just give her a call to see if she is a fit as a keynote speaker for your event or to train in your organization.

- You can learn more about Peggy's speaking schedule, topics and solutions for solid GROWTH by visiting her online at **www.peggybrockman.com**
- Like her page and connect with her on Facebook at **/10FeetFromTheEdge** or **/peggybrockman**
- Follow her on Twitter **@brockmanpeggy**
- Join her mailing list for her monthly "Dose of Vitamin P" newsletter by visiting her website at **www.peggybrockman.com.**

TAKE *the* Next Steps

VISIT HER WEBSITE
www.PeggyBrockman.com

Keynote SPEAKER:

BOOK PEGGY for your organization or event – topics customized to your needs.

Empowerment Mentoring TELESEMINAR PROGRAM:

If you enjoyed this book – you will LOVE this program! DISCOVER, TRANSFORM and ACHIEVE through 12 thought provoking, life changing, mentoring for success calls including topics like: Comfort Zone; Purpose, Vision & Goals; Perception; Authentic Journaling; Attitude; Forgiveness; Terror Barrier; Self-Belief and MORE. Calls recorded for your review and convenience.

Corporate TRAINING:

Personal and Professional Development; Leadership; Sales; Personality and Learning Styles; Customer Service; Values and many more! Programs customized to your company's needs.

Personal or GROUP COACHING:

Local in person; Long distance by Skype or Phone.

John Maxwell Leadership TRAINING PROGRAMS:

Becoming A Person Of Influence; Everyone Communicates Few Connect; How To Be A REAL Success; Put Your Dreams To The Test; The 21 Irrefutable Laws Of Leadership; Leadership Gold; The 15 Invaluable Laws of Growth and MORE!

The *Sales Alphabet* 13 Week WEBINAR TRAINING PROGRAM

An invaluable tool for your sales team as well as anyone in the network marketing or direct sales industry. Two lessons covered in each 90 minute weekly call. Calls recorded for review.

Other Mastermind groups and programs include:

As a Man Thinketh by James Allen

Discover Your Sweet Spot by Scott Fay

Re-Inventing YOU – A VIP Day for Women

Connect, Communicate and Close sales workshop
(Customized for specific sales groups like realtors, network marketers, media sales, etc.)

$\mathcal{A}$CKNOWLEDGEMENTS

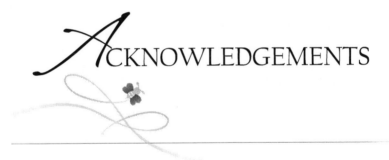

There are so many I would like to thank for helping make this book a reality. So many friends and family members that I can't acknowledge them all here – you know who you are.

BILL BROCKMAN

To my "for-life partner" – my husband – It took me a while to find you. We can call it fate, but God knew what he was doing. We have had some tough times and some beautiful times … that is life. As Bette Midler sings – *You Are The Wind Beneath My Wings*. You let me be me even when you don't understand why sometimes. You are my forever love.

BROOKLYN BIRCHFIELD

My first born – my angel I never thought possible. Your life has not always been easy. You are a survivor and you inspire me for being the woman you are. You know what it is to suffer with a debilitating disease – ulcerative colitis – that robs you of many things in life, yet you push through every day because that is who you are. You gave me one of the greatest gifts in life – my two beautiful and amazing grandsons – Sydian and Elijah. You gave me another gift when you took the chapters of my book and added more life to them through your innate word-smithing ability. You have such a sweet and beautiful soul and you are talented in so many ways. I love you to the moon and back.

CALLIE GARDINER

You were the best surprise of my life. You came only 11 ½ months after your sister. You were the sassy one and always so full of life and laughter. Your talents and insight amaze me. You have gifted so many with your artistic talent and brought the cover of my book to life with your incredible talent as a photographer. You too, have pushed through a debilitating disease. Mal de Debarquement Syndrome (MdDS) has robbed you of many things you love over the past year, yet you push through and still delight in making others laugh. I pray they one day find a cure or that it just disappears. Your deep sense of caring is a gift to all who know you. Thank you for bringing our British family, David and his two beautiful children, Janine and Craig, into our lives. No matter how old you are, you will always be my sassy little C-Boo whom I love so dearly. You are your mother's child.

TINA SEARS PROCHILO

You are my hero. In spite of all you experienced as a child and even as an adult, you are a survivor. God brought you into our life when you were only 17. We needed each other and always have. I am so blessed to be able to call you my daughter. I have always believed in the gift that you are and the talents you have. I hope that your sweet husband, Mark, and his beautiful daughter, Grace, truly appreciate the love you have to give. You took on the challenge of adult on-set Type 1 Diabetes and you didn't let it define you. You defined it and how you would take control of it. I am so proud of the woman you are. I love you.

JEANETTE FANCONI
and STACY BROCKMAN

You were two of the greatest gifts your father gave me. I am so blessed to be your "Mom." When you came into our family, I know you both thought we were a little crazy at first. You wondered what on earth your dad had gotten you all into. Then you discovered it was OK to step outside your comfort zone and act a little crazy; and even laugh so hard ice cream comes out your nose. Jeanette, you are a wonderful wife to Jason and mother to our two precious grandsons, Evan and Brock. You have always been way too self-sufficient but I know you know we are here for you. Stacy, you were so shy and insecure when we first met. Like a butterfly, I watched you break through your cocoon and blossom into a beautiful woman. The story of learning to drive might sound very familiar to you! I love you both and I am so proud of you.

LISA BERRYHILL DAVIS

We have been through so much together. Business partners at one time, best friends for over 25 years, we have shared moments most people would never believe! I was there for the birth of your child and you have been there for my girls through the years. It was you and your talents as a writer yourself that helped me get "unstuck" and move forward with this book. You helped me to see what I needed to do to re-order my chapters and to open it with a more powerful start. Through the years, we have always had each other. I love you girl and I can't wait to read your first book. I know it is coming soon.

JOYCE SANDERS

You have been my mentor, my dearest friend, and one of my "Twisted Sisters" for so many years now. I wouldn't be where I am today without your encouragement and wisdom. You have an incredible ability to make people laugh. You are always there for me with your encouraging words, a listening ear and your talent for seeing the bigger picture. Even when we are apart, we know we are only a phone call away — and there have been a lot of those phone hours! I will never go into Winn Dixie again or eat ice cream without thinking of you … and smiling. I love you my friend – thank you for taking this journey with me and celebrating each step along the way.

To all my other *"Twisted Sisters"*
MY GIRLFRIEND GROUP
I am so blessed to have you in my life. We will be there for each other through thick and thin. Marnie Tate, your acts of kindness are never overlooked and always so appreciated. You are a shining light with a beautiful spirit and an amazing connector; Vickie Warner, I owe you sister! I value your friendship so much. I look so forward to being able to spend more time together and making more memories now that you are retired; Jan Pooley, you give so much to so many, I am blessed to call you friend; Jeanne Rief, you are a true friend and we have shared so many special moments together. I love you all. And in case you have forgotten - I will always be the youngest!

BARBARA JONES *and* BARBARA BRITT
Thank you for taking the time to completely read my book midway and then again in its "almost final" format. You shared your insight to help make it complete. B.Jones, we meet people who become woven into our lives in a very special way. At times we have been miles and even years apart yet you've always been there as my friend for over 30 years. You have given me so many great gifts in life. Your peace work in non-violent communication is a gift to many across the world. B.Britt, my newest friend and partner on the John Maxwell Team, our journey has just begun. We will have many years together of

changing people's lives for the better through our speaking, training and coaching. I am blessed to have you in my life.

BARRY SMITH *and* SUSAN YOUNG

My coaching partners – you both inspired and encouraged me in so many ways. You are both talented authors, speakers and coaches and I know we will all ROCK THIS WORLD in our own special ways. Barry, you were one of the first to read my beginning chapters and gave me great direction on what was "missing." Susan, you inspire me with your desire to serve and your infectious energy and talent. I am blessed to have you both in my life.

MY JOHN MAXWELL TEAM MENTORS

Paul Martinelli, YOU are an amazing man! You have taught me so much by just observing you in action and listening to you speak and train. You give so much to so many. The members of the John Maxwell Team are blessed by your leadership and mentorship. **Scott Fay**, you inspired me and touched my heart the first time I connected with you. I am proud of you for *Discover Your Sweet Spot.* Your book will inspire many and I will enjoy offering it as a Mastermind group. **Ed DeCosta**, I just like you - you are right on. You tell it like it is and hold people accountable. **Christian Simpson**, I learned so much about something I love, being a coach, from the hours of video and audio training I spent with you. You are brilliant! **Roddy Galbraith**, what a gift you are with your expert knowledge of what a real speaker is and does. The Empowerment Mentoring program you, Paul and Les Brown created is changing lives daily and I am proud to be a facilitator of it. **Melissa West,**

you WOW me with your energy, your enthusiasm and your tambourines! Your WOW book will be a big success.

JOHN C. MAXWELL

I have followed you for almost 20 years and am so proud to be a part of your speaking, training and coaching team to help carry on your legacy. Thank you for the gift of spending a week with you in Guatemala on our transformational leadership mission trip. It was truly life changing as you will see in Chapter 11 of my book. YOU INSPIRE ME!

KENDRA CAGLE, JULIE ESCOBAR *and* KELLY HUMPHREY

YOU GIRLS ROCK! You made my book come to life through your talents in graphics, words and editing. Your final touches were just what it needed to POP!

Last, but certainly not least...

MAMA AND DADDY

Celine Dion summed it up perfectly in the lyrics to her song *Because You Loved Me.*

> For all those times you stood by me
> For all the truth that you made me see
> For all the joy you brought to my life
> For all the wrong that you made right
> For every dream you made come true

You have been my strength, my voice at times and you saw the best there was in me. I am everything I am because you loved me. THANK YOU will never be enough. I love you.

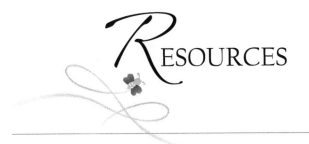

RESOURCES

If you or someone you know suffers from ulcerative colitis or other colorectal diseases, there are some organizations that could be helpful.

The longest standing and most noted of these is **The Ostomy Association of America.**

Their website is located at **www.ostomy.org.**

There, you will be able to find information about many types of ostomy surgery. You can also locate a chapter nearest you.

If you are interested in learning more about the internal Kock Pouch or BCIR surgery, here are a couple of websites I have used.

http://bcir.com/ is the site of the Continent Ostomy Center at Palms of Pasadena Hospital in St. Petersburg, Florida where I had my Kock Pouch revised to a BCIR in 1998 and where I also had some hernia repairs.

http://ileostomy-surgery.com/ and **http://www.kockpouch.com/** are both Dr. Don Schiller's sites. He is a surgeon in Los Angeles, California I have used and really like.

I have also visited with a surgeon who does the Kock Pouch procedure at Ochsner Health System, a hospital in New Orleans, Louisiana. There are a limited number of surgeons who do the Kock Pouch or BCIR surgery and I like to know who they are in each direction if there was ever an emergency while I am traveling. It is something that gives me control in knowing that they know my history and could treat me if needed. It also gives me choices.

Do your research on the Ileo-anal anastomosis – or J-Pouch – surgery as well. This is another type of pouch surgery that offers a popular choice if the rectum can remain intact.

If you are considering ostomy surgery, do your research and talk with several people before you make a final decision. Unfortunately, many surgeons who only do the standard Brooke Ileostomy will not tell you about the other options out there or they will tell you they are not good options. Do what is best for you. It is your life and your choice. There can be complications with any type of surgery and the complications I had were not because I had the internal pouch surgery. There were many factors involved.

Don't wait until it is an emergency to make a decision if you don't have to. You will give the power of choice to someone else. If you have a Brooke Ileostomy and are interested in having an internal pouch, talk with doctors who do that surgery to see if it is an option for you. I have had both. I love the internal pouch but I would accept the external bag if I had to go back to it. It would just be another "new normal."

Make the

MOST

of your

Journey;

the

ALTERNATIVE

is NOT a good option!

Made in the USA
Charleston, SC
15 September 2014